CHILD GROWTH

Ann Arbor
Science
Library

131
K74
1972

Child Growth

by *Wilton Marion Krogman*

ANN ARBOR
THE UNIVERSITY OF MICHIGAN PRESS

PREFACE

This book is the fruit of some forty years of research in, and interpretation of, the physical growth of the human child. I have studied child growth in Cleveland, Chicago, and Philadelphia, and have been privileged to be affiliated with other child research units, either as associate or as consultant.

In the pages that follow I have covered quite a range of biological and behavioral growth-patterns, discussing both intrinsic factors (as genetics, endocrines) and extrinsic factors (as nutrition, socio-economic variables). I have, wherever applicable, drawn upon my own researches, essentially in the biological (morphological) areas. I have, as necessary, drawn freely upon the studies of others; work either correlative with mine, or in the broader fields of behavioral and adaptive unfolding. I have not burdened the pages with detailed citations or references to professional journals. I have given names of both researchers and research units whenever specific items are referred to. At the end of this book I have given a selected number of useful, more general references.

I am indebted to publishers of books and journals and to authors for permission to reproduce the illustrations in this book. Acknowledgments are given on pages 223–24.

If this book is read with the joy and satisfaction with which it was researched and written, I shall be pleased.

WILTON MARION KROGMAN
Lancaster, Pennsylvania

CONTENTS

INTRODUCTION

Evolution and Human Growth

Three billion years ago—within a few million years plus or minus—life appeared on the Earth. It probably began from some combination of the basic and universal CHON —carbon, hydrogen, oxygen, nitrogen. In time, a protein molecule came into being, the building-block of life as we know it. But, it was a "self-replicating macromolecule" —a giant molecule that could reproduce itself, life begetting life. Thus, growth also came into being, for intrinsically, growth and life are synonymous, life being the spark, and growth the time-limited flame. Viewed in such perspective, growth becomes both phylogenetic—the evolutionary and progressive unfolding of *all* life—and ontogenetic—the development of the life-form of each *individual* within a specific group.

Evolution's long road to man has passed many milestones: first unicellular, then multicellular; first simple, then complex; first generalized, then specialized; first invertebrate, then vertebrate; and finally the progression from fish to amphibian to mammal. It is no wonder, therefore, that the human growth pattern has in it much that is vertebrate, much that is mammalian, much that is primate (man's simian nearest-of-kin), and relatively very little that is specifically human.

Organic growth, in all of its aspects, encompasses the entire life-span, prenatal and postnatal, of each individual living organism. In order to demonstrate how man shares in this organic growth process, and how his is a modified and adapted pattern, it is necessary to set up a rather arbitrary dichotomy: 1) the period of growth, per se; 2) the period of age-changes.

In the discussion that follows I shall accept the human postnatal growth period as twenty years. By then all long-bone growth has ceased. After this we speak of age-changes at cellular and tissue or systemic level. For the most part growth and age-changes are progressive, cumulative, and irreversible.

Man has absolutely the most protracted period of infancy, childhood, and juvenility of all forms of life, i.e., he is a *neotenous* or long-growing animal. Nearly thirty per cent of his entire life-span is devoted to growing. This long-drawn-out growth period is distinctively human; it makes of man a learning, rather than a purely instinctive, animal. Man is programmed to *learn* to behave, rather than to react via an imprinted determinative instinctual code. Or, to put it another way, the human child has *both* a biological and a cultural inheritance, rather than only a biological.

In this total biocultural growth complex there are four major aspects of growth to be considered:

1. *Motor growth,* which involves gross body control plus finer motor coordination. It runs the gamut of all bodily movements and postural responses, such as head-balance, creeping, sitting, standing, walking, prehensility, grasp, and manipulation.

2. *Adaptive responses,* involving the neuromuscular coordination of the entire body, such as eye-hand coordination. Strictly speaking, the adaptive responses involve the use of the body's entire motor equipment directed to the performance of a specific task.

3. *Language,* which includes all forms of communication, ranging from bodily movements, facial expressions,

to vocalization. Language, which involves symbolism, is learned early, but abstract thinking is said not to begin until considerably later (some say as late as twelve years).

4. *Personal-social development and adjustment.* This is the sum of the child's reaction to the environment. It involves both an intrinsic (biological) and extrinsic (cultural) reaction to stimuli. The child is first an organic entity then an interacting being at a personal-social level.

Each in its own sphere—the biological and the cultural —has been well and thoughtfully researched. Unfortunately the research has often been of an either-or kind, i.e., either physical growth alone, or behavioral unfolding alone, has been tackled. But correlated studies in both major spheres—on the same group of children—are embarrassingly few.

Varieties of Growth and Development

The term "growth" and "development" are often used interchangeably. Strictly speaking they are not interchangeable. *Growth* refers to proportionate changes in size, *development* to increasing complexity (e.g., the formation of the four-chambered fetal heart from the straight pulsating tube of the embryo) and progress toward maturity. Both processes are integrative, with growth perhaps somewhat more structural, development more functional, with the structure preceding function.

At the risk of oversimplification it is possible to set up three aspects of human growth and development: 1) we grow; 2) we grow up; 3) we grow older. Let us look at these in order.

1. *We grow.* This is *size*. With but few exceptions (e.g., the thymus, the circumference of the dental arches) every dimension of the human body gets larger with age during the prenatal period and the first two decades of the postnatal period.

2. *We grow up.* This is *proportion.* We grow at different rates, at different times, in different areas, systems, or

organs of the body. Here is an over-all formula for the postnatal growth of the human body: 2–3–4–5, or, head and neck dimensions increase by two times, trunk by three times, arm by four times, leg by five times. Thus, via a time-integrated process, a newborn baby becomes an adult.

3. *We grow older.* This is *maturation.* Every tissue in the body bears an indelible register of the passage of biological time. In this sense maturation is a process, maturity is a goal. Nature's goals are two: 1) sexual or reproductive maturity; 2) adult or species-stable maturity. (In a later chapter we shall develop the theme of maturation.)

In addition to growth changes in size and proportion and shape, there are other changes that man undergoes. There are changes in *kind,* or the appearance and disappearance of different kinds of cells, tissues, and organs, as for example the three primordial embryonic layers of ectoderm, mesoderm, and endoderm, and their derivatives. There are changes in *number,* from the single cell at fertilization to the sixty trillion cells of the adult of twenty years. There are changes in *position,* for example the prenatal migration of the diaphragm from a neck-level (fourth cervical level) to an abdominal level (twelfth thoracic or first lumbar level), or the eruptional migration of the teeth in the jaws. There are changes in *composition,* as changes in pigmentation of eye and skin with age, or changes of body-water content (ninety per cent in the fetus, seventy-three per cent in the newborn, sixty per cent at one year of age). There are changes in growth-*timing,* which are genetic or species-linked; for example, in the anthropoid the first permanent molar tooth erupts at about three years of age, while in man it is "the six-year molar." There are changes in *body-build* (so-called "constitution" or "body type") ranging from the linear or slender to the lateral or stocky, with an intermediate athletic or muscular build. This, by the way, is a very important growth change to keep in mind, for it means differing height-weight ratios for the growing body-builds. A slender-build child may be expected to weigh less for his height than a stocky-build child of comparable age, sex, ethnic background, and so on.

Patterns of Systemic Growth

In the 1920's, Prof. Richard Scammon of the University of Minnesota reduced the growth curves of the human body to four basic "curves of systemic or organic growth," for both prenatal and postnatal growth. At this point only the postnatal curves will be considered. The curves are based on the principle that at age twenty years all dimensional sizes are adult and have one hundred per cent of their value, starting at birth with zero per cent. For each year, then, each curve has a certain percentage of its adult value. Scammon proposed four systemic curves: neural, general, lymphoid, genital (Figure 1).

1. *Neural,* which includes the brain and cord and their coverings, the entire optic apparatus, and the related bony parts of the skull, the upper face, and the vertebral column. This curve is truly remarkable, for it has a tremendous velocity, i.e., the curve rises steeply upwards and to the right. I have always been impressed by the significance of this curve: by about the age of seven or eight years (the age of school beginning) the brain has nearly ninety-five per cent of its adult size; it is practically adult in size, shape, convolutionary pattern (the gyri and sulci or folds and furrows), and cytoarchetectonic structure (the interrelations of all nerve pathways within the brain). By the age of seven or eight years the child has about all the brain mass—the "raw stuff"—that he ever will have. I am tempted to give here a biological definition of education: teaching and learning are the translation of capacity or potential into ability; Nature says, in effect, "here's a brain ready in about the first grade, to receive instruction." Then, since the human childhood is long,

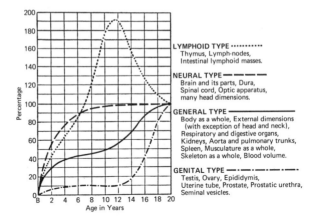

FIG. 1. The Four Basic Curves of Postnatal Growth.

may follow the eight years of elementary school, the four of high school, and on into the college years.

2. *General,* which includes the external dimensions of the body as a whole (except the bony housing of the brain, the eye, and the spinal cord). Here are included the respiratory, vascular, and digestive systems, the skeleton, the musculature, and kidney and bladder. This curve has a high velocity (steep upward curve) to about five years, then a relative plateau to about ten or eleven years, then another upsweep, and a final slowed-down attainment of adult size. This curve is often called "sigmoid"— a rough S-curve, lying on its side, so to speak. Since this general curve really encompasses almost all of the human body I have renamed it the *Body Curve*—for *b*one, *b*rawn, *b*lood, *b*reathing, *b*owel, and *b*ladder (i.e., the urinary portion of the urino-genital system).

3. *Lymphoid,* which includes the thymus, the lymph nodes of the body, and the intestinal lymphatic masses (including the appendix). This is an interesting curve for it rises to a crescendo of two hundred per cent, sometime between ten and fifteen years of age, i.e., we then have twice as much lymphoid material as we do as adults. The

scale-down from two hundred to one hundred per cent is mainly achieved by the involution of the thymus which loses much of its secretory function and reverts to connective tissue.

4. *Genital,* which includes the primary sex apparatus and all secondary sex traits. Here are the gonads (ovary in female, testis in male) and all structures associated with reproductive sex. The curve has a small upturn in the first year of life and is then quiescent until sometime near and after ten years of age. It then literally explodes into the dynamic upturn that marks the circum-pubertal growth acceleration—the time during which the child "grows like a weed," "shoots up," and so on.

I think it is important, at this point, to observe that these four curves are characteristic of the human kind, *Homo sapiens.* The curves are so basic that it is reasonable to conclude that they are genetically entrenched with equal vigor in *all children the world over.* If there are so-called "racial" differences they are essentially environmental, not genetic. We shall come back to this problem in later chapters.

Some Methodological Principles

It is time, now, to turn to a discussion of some of the methodological principles that will be employed in this volume. First of all, we shall not be plagued with involved statistical procedures. For our purposes the mean or average, the normal range of variation or standard deviation, the percentile ranking, and the coefficient of correlation will suffice. These are presented in Appendix I.

There are two major ways in which to secure growth data: 1) cross-sectional; 2) longitudinal or serial. The *cross-sectional* method is an early one and yields only general information on growth. It is based on differing samples at each age—for example, one hundred boys or girls at birth, another one hundred at one year, another one hundred at two years, and so on. The mean and standard deviation of each sample are calculated, tabulated, and graphed. Hence, over-all population sampling may be done in a relatively short time.

The *longitudinal* or *serial* method is more recent, and is based upon the regular, follow-up observation of a sample of the same children—at birth, three months, six, nine, twelve, eighteen, twenty-four months and every six months to five years, and every year thereafter to 20:0. The data accruing from this kind of study will tell how *each child grows as an individual* in height, weight, or any dimension or proportion we wish to observe.

Cross-sectional data, when applied to a child, will tell where he or she stands with reference to other children. Longitudinal data on that child will tell where he or she stands with reference to his or her own progress in growth and in maturational development. When at my Growth Center I first see a child I evaluate stature, for example, for *status* and *comparability*, using cross-sectional tabulations. Then, after I have seen the child four or five times (in, say, a two-year period) I can evaluate *progress* and *family-line* relationship. Then, with all four of these criteria in proper context, I can grant the child the growth *individuality* that is his or her birthright.

An individual child's growth pattern should not be judged by a moment of time—at 6:0, at 10:0, at 14:0—but rather in time-depth, observing progress rather than status.

The word "progress" is the key to the realization that there are several *stages* of growth between birth and twenty years. There is a periodicity in growth which is a matter of relative speed (fast period, slow period) and area or region, leading to differential growth (a time, for example, of height gain, or of weight gain; or of head-face growth and of arm-leg growth). The basic idea is, simply, that the child does not grow "all-of-a-piece," expanding, as it were, radially from some central point.

The Classification of Postnatal Growth-Periods

There are a number of well-defined "way stations" in postnatal growth. There are times of fast growth and of slowed-down growth. There are times of greater or lesser integrative complexity. We do not follow, in a uniform even progression, but rather an irregular progression, as relates to timing and extent of change. The classification that I have found the most useful is as follows:

Period	*Male*	*Female*
I. Infancy (neonate)	Birth–1 year (1st 2 weeks)	Birth–1 year (1st 2 weeks)
II. Childhood	1–16 years	1–15 years
early	1– 6 years	1– 6 years
mid	6 to 9–10 years	6 to 9–10 years
late	9–10 to 16 years	9–10 to 15 years
III. Puberty (in late childhood)	13–14 years	12–13 years
IV. Adolescence	14 to 18–20 years	13 to 18–20 years
V. Adult	20 years +	20 years +

This breakdown of age-periods is not an arbitrary one, for it is based on *major* changes in growth tempo and growth integration. The *neonate* period of two weeks registers the adjustive time-period of being born: by ten to fourteen days the babe has regained his birth weight. The *infancy* period of the first postnatal year is, perhaps, the most important single growth-year of all: birth weight has tripled and length has increased by one-half; the brain is growing at a tremendous rate; the teeth are forming (the milk teeth have begun to erupt and most of the permanent teeth have begun to calcify in their sockets in the jaws); the whole learning period is well launched. In very fact the first postnatal growth year sets both pace and direction.

Childhood lasts a long time, biologically speaking. The *early* period, up to age six years, sees the baby teeth all erupted and in good working order; brain growth is nearly done; language is well along, as is the socialization process; the child is basically family-oriented, but peer-grouping has begun. *Mid*-childhood is sort of an interim period; the current of growth has slowed down so that size gain is minimal; by the age of nine years or so the child's body proportions foreshadow those of the adult; brain growth is through; the replacement of baby teeth with permanent teeth is well under way; learning proceeds evenly, not too rapidly: The second five years of postnatal growth-time is a period of consolidation: gains made are stabilized, are slowly advanced, and are firmly entrenched. But mid-childhood is literally a calm before a storm! *Late* child-hood is a time of vigorous growth and seismic change. At ten to twelve years or so the "adolescent growth spurt" sweeps in—the most rapid growth since the birth-one year period; it is during this time that the boy becomes a man, the girl becomes a woman, for *puberty* occurs, with its profound morphological, biochemical, and psychological changes. Even though I give averages (thirteen to four-teen years for boys, twelve to thirteen years for girls) the normal range is *any time* in late childhood. In late child-hood all permanent teeth up to and including second molar have erupted.

It will be noted that I put *adolescence,* as a period, *after* puberty, even though the so-called "adolescent growth spurt" begins prepubertally. I personally regard adolescence as more of a behavioral than a biological phenomenon. It is a becoming-used-to period, a time of adjustment and understanding comprehension; it is be-tween the achievement of sexuality and the threshold of adult responsibility; it is a role-learning period. Someone has said of a late "teener" that he is a "part-time adult."

Adult? Well, twenty years is a logical terminal growth-age. Body size, from skeleton to all other organ systems, is definitive. There may be a little growth in the total vertebral column, adding about a half inch to stature, but the half-inch gain will be in sitting height, not in long bones of the leg.

There are age-period classifications, other than the one above discussed, for both European and American children. These I have brought together and tabulated in Appendix II.

PRENATAL DEVELOPMENT
AND THE
NEWBORN CHILD

Growth of the Embryo and Fetus

Prenatal growth and development in man is a process shared by all mammals. Starting with an ovum fertilized by a sperm there are six definable stages:

Prenatal Stage	*Changes Which Occur*
1. Cleavage	Growth begins via cell division
2. Implantation of ovum	Fertilized egg attached to uterine wall; growth rate is speeded-up because of improved nutrition
3. Formation of germ layers	Three basic cell layers: ectoderm, mesoderm, endoderm; growth is organized and differentiated
4. Formation of organs of the embryo	Nerve tube, body somites, limb buds, etc., are formed; differential growth times and velocities established
5. Adult organ formation	Embryonic organs are transformed via tissue formation; nerve tracts established
6. Fetal development	Appearance of more organized motor behavior: nervous stimulation results in behavioral patterns

The three cell layers of Stage 3 give rise to all tissues, organs, and structures which characterize the human child. Their basic derivatives are as follows:

ECTODERM	MESODERM	ENDODERM

1. Skin
 cutaneous glands
 hair, nails
 lens of eye
 2. Epithelium of
 sense organs
 nasal cavity
 sinuses
 mouth
   oral glands
   enamel (teeth)
 anal canal
 3. Nervous tissue, in-
 cluding pituitary
 and chromaffin
 tissue
	1. All types muscle
	 2. Connective tis-
	 sue, cartilage,
	 bone, notochord
	 3. Blood, bone
	 marrow
	 4. Lymphoid tissue
	 5. Epithelium of
	 blood vessels
	 lymphatics
	   body cavities
	 kidney, ureter
	 gonads, genital
	 ducts
	 adrenal cortex
	 joint cavities
		1. Epithelium of
		 pharynx
		   root of tongue
		 auditory tube
		 tonsils
		 thyroid
		 parathyroid
		 thymus
		 2. Larynx, trachea,
		 lungs
		 3. Digestive tube
		 and associated
		 glands
		 4. Bladder
		 5. Vagina (all?)
		 vestibule
		 6. Urethra and
		 associated glands

Growth is intrinsically at cellular level; such growth is of three major types, as this schema demonstrates (after Williams and Wendell-Smith, 1966).

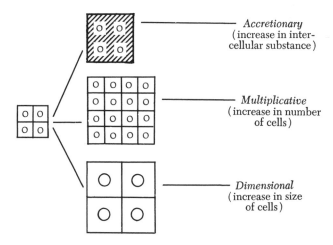

Accretionary (increase in inter- cellular substance)

Multiplicative (increase in number of cells)

Dimensional (increase in size of cells)

(these go on more or less simultaneously)

Assume that we start with four cells: they may grow by *accretion,* or increase in the amount of intercellular material; by *multiplication,* or increase in the number of cells; and *dimensional,* or increase in cell size. These three processes, integratively, result in embryonic and fetal growth.

The rate of prenatal growth is almost beyond belief. The ovum has a maximum diameter of 0.2 mm, and a volume of 0.004 ($\pm$) mm; it weighs 0.004 mg, and when the sperm enters it, 0.005 mg. A full-term male infant weighs 3,250 gms, hence, weight increase from ovum to birth is 65 billion per cent! It has been calculated that if the growth *rate* of the first postconceptual month be continued until the twentieth postnatal year the resultant mass would be $(128,350)^{1100 \text{ light years}}$ across (about the size of the known universe and expanding peripherally with nearly the speed of light).

Tremendous rate of growth is also seen in the first postnatal year, during which birth length is increased by fifty per cent, birth weight by two hundred per cent. If *this rate* were to continue until the child reached adulthood he would be over 1,150 feet tall and weigh nearly fifty million pounds!

Obviously, the prenatal growth rate decelerates as term is approached and after the child is born. For example, the postnatal weight-growth rate is 25.7% in the first month, 6.2% by the sixth month, and 1.9% by the twelfth month.

In terms of absolute size here are a few comparisons: at ten days of age the embryo is the size of a pinhead; at three weeks the size of an apple seed; at four weeks the size of a grape; at five weeks the size of a walnut; at six weeks the size of a golf ball; at two months the size of a hen's egg; at five months the fetus weighs 1¼ pounds; at six months, 2¼ pounds; at eight months 4¼ pounds; and the full-term newborn weights 7–7½ pounds.

When the child is born there is a temporary reversal in

one aspect of growth, i.e., in weight. In the first ten days of postnatal life the average weight loss is 7.1%; during this ten-day period the average weight loss is least for first born, next for second-fourth born, most for fifth + born. About twenty-six per cent of all babies regain their birth weight by the end of the first week. There is said to be a seasonal difference: babies born in summer and autumn get back to their birth weight in ten days, but winter-spring babies return to only about ninety-five per cent of birth weight.

Structural and Behavioral Changes

In very early prenatal life—when the organism is about one inch long—overt behavior has its inception; it is "behavior" in a purely morphological sense, but there is some reason to feel that such early behavioral reactions may foreshadow certain later prenatal and even postnatal behavioral patterns. The total prenatal behavioral pattern is genetically entrenched, certainly at species level (this includes all human children), possibly at body-build and/or familial level (inheritance within family-lines, both maternal and paternal).

It is impossible here to go into a literal day-by-day account. However, I venture to offer a sketchy timetable of certain embryo-fetus *structural* changes; time is expressed as related to the week *after* last menstruation (adapted from Arey, 1954):

Age in weeks	*Structural changes*
2–3 (EMBRYO)	fertilization; egg down tube to uterus; cell division initiated
4–5	implantation in uterine wall; skeleton and nervous system begin to develop
6–7	head, heart, tail visible; chest and abdomen formed; limbs and eyes develop; gill pouch vestiges seen; length 6–12 mm ($\frac{1}{4}''$–$\frac{1}{2}''$)

Age in weeks (cont.)	*Structural changes* (cont.)
8–9 (FETUS)	face fully developed and is "human"; gill vestiges go; length 21–30 mm ($\frac{7}{8}''$–$1\frac{1}{8}''$), weight 1–2 gms ($\frac{1}{28}$–$\frac{1}{14}$ oz)
14	limbs, including nails, completely formed; external genitals recognizable; 77 mm ($3''$), 30 gms (1 oz)
18	"quickening" movements; heart beat audible; 190 mm ($8\frac{1}{2}''$), 180 gms ($6\frac{1}{2}$ oz)

After this the story is one of general fetal growth in size and improvement in viability. At twenty-seven weeks the eyes open; at thirty-two weeks the fetus is 400 mm ($16''$), 1425 gms (3 lbs, 2 oz), and, if given special care, is viable. At thirty-six weeks with length 450 mm ($18''$) and weight 2375 gms (5 lbs, 4 oz) chances of survival are good (better in eighth month than in seventh). At forty weeks comes *term,* at 500 mm ($20''$) and 3250 gms (7 lbs, 4 oz).

The earliest, if not the first, behavioral reaction is in the mouth-neck area. At the eighth week, upon oral stimulation, the body bends unilaterally, and at the tenth week bilaterally. In the eleventh week the fingers flex (they "clasp"). In the twelfth week the hands approximate one another as though to "patty-cake." At this time the arm is raised, hand goes to mouth, and sucking movements may occur;* the controlateral (opposite) hand contracts. At fourteen weeks the facial muscles contract in a "sneer," accompanied by swallowing movements; the eyes wink, though eyelids are still fused. At sixteen weeks there is a single shallow gasp.

Between twelve and sixteen weeks almost all of the skin of the body surface reacts to stimulus. The head can move independently of the trunk (it can rotate, tilt, and retract). The eyeballs move, the eyelids blink; the lips

*Babies have been born with callused hands/fingers due to constant sucking *in utero.*

protrude (the upper, a day or so before the lower); the mouth opens and closes, with definite swallowing motions. Arms and legs show relatively independent movements, even at joints (simulation of locomotion?). There are exhalatory chest movements.

In the eighteenth week the fingers have a firm grip. In twenty weeks the whole arm is extended laterally, the head turning to the side of extension. In twenty-two weeks there is a grouped series of respiratory gasps, continued to the twenty-fifth week as continuous prerespiratory chest movements. At twenty-six weeks the fetus is viable, able to breathe.

The development of the *senses* is of interest. Taste buds appear at the third month, and at birth the child can distinguish sweet from sour, bitter, and salt. The olfactory and tactile areas of the brain are among the earliest to be myelinated (sheathing for functional use). In all probability, however, there is no adequate smell stimulus in prenatal life. Hearing does not become effective until early postnatal life (the onset of breathing opens the Eustachian tube and drains the middle ear). Cellular changes leading to eye formation begin in the second-third embryonic week, but binocular vision, visual space perception, and stereo-perception develop postnatally. The newborn baby shows evidence of light sensitivity in a light-stimulated pupillary reflex.

I want to disgress here a moment to mention one very important structural growth adaptation in the human growth pattern. I have said earlier that man is a mammal. This is true. But he is a special kind of mammal—he is an upright mammal (a biped), not an all-fours mammal (a quadruped). Even so, the basic human growth pattern is mammalian. In the quadrupeds, bodily growth has three main gradients or directions: head to tail, back to front, and mid-line to lateral; in us, as bipeds, these directions are, respectively, superior-inferior or vertical, posterior-anterior or sagittal, and mid-line to lateral or transverse. This type of growth analysis in the developing child is extremely useful in understanding the "streams" of functional growth; the arms and legs in directional sequence; outward or laterally from the trunk in the embryo and fetus.* When the postnatal growth of head and face is studied the craniofacial heights, breadths, and depths (lengths) grow exactly as in the mammalian body.

The prenatal period is terminated by birth—by the first breath of the newborn baby. It is a complex integration of morphological, physiological, and biochemical changes, the full interrelations of which are not fully understood. Robert Frost commented on the sudden thawing of snow on a sunny hillside:

> *As often as I've seen it done before,*
> *I can't pretend to tell the way it's done.*

So, too, we may epitomize the miracle of birth.

Premature Birth

I heard my first lecture in obstetrics over forty-five years ago. I vividly remember the words of the teacher: "Ladies and gentlemen, the miracle is not of birth, but of birth *almost* perfect." He then went on to discuss structure and function of the full-term baby with relation to norms and variability. Next, he stated that "full-term" meant forty weeks or ten lunar months (ten months of four weeks or twenty-eight days each, for a total of two hundred and eighty days). Then arises the question of the baby born *before* the stated forty-week full-term standard.

The Premature Infant

Classically the prematurely born child has been defined as follows: 1) born between 28th-37th weeks of gestation;

*Arms and legs, as they grow out from the trunk, develop their own gradient in terms of developmental timing. In both it is peripheral to central: in the arm it is hand-forearm-upper arm-shoulder; in the leg it is foot-lower leg-thigh-pelvis.

2) birth weight 2500 gms (5 lbs, 8 oz) or less; 3) birth length 47 cm (18½″) or less; 4) head length below 11.5 cm (4½″) and head circumference below 33 cm (13″); 5) chest circumference 30 cm (11¾″) or less; 6) disproportion between the head circumference/chest circumference ratio, which in full-term infants is about 93–100%, but in premature infants is as low as 83–85%.

The frequency of prematurity (under 37 wks.) is 7.6% in the U.S., 6.5% in England, 5.5% in Sweden, 7.0% in France, 10% in Japan, and 35% in one area of India where the average birth weight is only six pounds. The low birth weight baby bears a many-factored relationship to the maternal host: more frequent in primipara below twenty or over forty years of age; commoner where mother's stature is below five feet; more often in unwed mothers because of the psycho-social emotionalism involved; frequent where the mother has had to work hard, physically, or for long hours, related in large part to other aspects of the lower socio-economic stratum; more often where maternal heart volume is below 50 (milliliters); where the mother has a history of difficulty in "carrying a child to term." Cigarette smoking is considered by some to be a causative agent, for the frequency of prematurity is said to rise from 7.06% in those who smoke one to five cigarettes daily to 33.3% in those who smoke over thirty-one cigarettes daily.

Far too often prematurity is defined almost exclusively on a time-basis, i.e., less than thirty-seven weeks. Hence to say that such-and-such a percentage of prematures survive is not very meaningful. The chances of survival are differential if the prematures are grouped by birthweight, ranging from ninety-five per cent in those of weight 2000–2500 gms, down to ten to fifteen per cent in those of weight 1000 gms, or less. Survival gains, due to modern research and detailed analysis, have more than doubled the chances of the < 1000 gms group.

Premature infants not only regain lost birth weight in

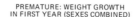

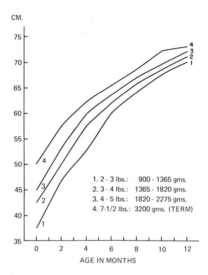

PREMATURE: WEIGHT GROWTH
IN FIRST YEAR (SEXES COMBINED)

1. 2 - 3 lbs.:   900 - 1365 gms.
2. 3 - 4 lbs.:   1365 - 1820 gms.
3. 4 - 5 lbs.:   1820 - 2275 gms.
4. 7-1/2 lbs.: 3200 gms. (TERM)

FIG. 2. Weight Gain in Premature Babies in the First Postnatal Year.

the first ten days more slowly, but their total postnatal growth rate is less. Once more, however, we must consider the evidence by birth-weight categories. In Figure 2, weight gain is shown in three groups of premature infants as compared to the full-term infant. The curves are, over-all, much alike, and are, as expected, in order from smallest birth-weight to normal. In Figure 3 the same birth-weight grouping is done for birth-one year growth in head circumference. Here the three groups of low-weight newborns catch up to one another, but *none* attain the full-term value.

The postnatal growth of the premature child has been summarized by Watson and Lowrey (1967) but the data cited are not always clearly defined and the results not always comparable. Several pediatricians feel that there was some early postnatal catch-up growth, for it is stated that the *rate* of growth in prematures exceeded the nor-

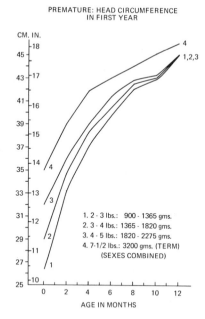

FIG. 3. Head Circumference in Premature Babies in the First Post-natal Year.

mal child in the birth-two year period. Pediatricians of Chicago concluded that prematures were the equivalent of norms by eight to ten years. A Swedish pediatrician stated that at puberty prematurely born children had the same height and weight as normals. On the other hand where the birth weight was under 1500 gms the children were still well below H-W norms at ten years of age. Baltimore prematurely born children, in a 1961 report, were still significantly underweight at six-seven years.

In an area of the most rapid growth—the head—the circumference in the premature babe has caught up to the norm of one year. Further, the head circumference/chest circumference proportion is nearly normal by six months after birth in moderately prematures who are responding optimally to postbirth care.

Premature birth is not the threat to postnatal growth and development that it once was. The data in the literature suggest that 1950 represented a major focal point of advance in knowledge of causes and their remedial treatment.

Congenital Failures

There is a rule called *The Bergonie-Tribondeau Law:* "Sensitivity of cells [to damage] varies directly with their reproductive capacity and inversely with their degree of differentiation." In principle this may be taken as applicable to the interpretation of the causes of congenital or birth defects; the interpretation centers around the *time* of prenatal (embryonic) development. In Figure 4 is a schematic drawing of the "sensitive" time period, related to embryonic length: 3.5 to 10 mm, in length, twenty-five to forty days after conception. If something goes wrong

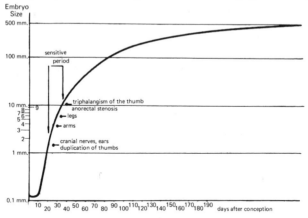

FIG. 4. The "Sensitive" Period in Early Embryonic Development.

in these particular fifteen days then the development of this embryo will be interfered with. Earliest to be affected will be certain cranial nerves, often those to the extrinsic muscles of the eyeball (i.e., those that permit eye movements), along with ear damage and an extra thumb (prepollex); a bit later arms and legs are hit; then the thumb again, with three, instead of the usual two, finger bones (phalanges), along with failure of the opening of the lower end of the intestines (rectum and anus are imperforate). These structures—even though they are un-related—are all liable to damage because they are being differentiated and/or formed or structured during this 25–40 day period. Tissue or organ vulnerability is thus a matter of critical *timing*.

The timing of thalidomide (a tranquilizing drug) dam-age is a bit different. Here the sensitive period is 34–50 days: 1) between days 34–38 the external ear is affected (no external ear or only a vestige), plus cranial nerves III, IV, VI, (muscles of the eyeball) and cranial nerve VII (to the facial muscles); between days 39–44 ($\pm$) the arm is malformed; between days 42–45 the leg is mal-formed (called phocomelia, for legs are fused and look seal-like); at or near day 50 the thumb has an extra phalanx and occasional anorectal imperforation occurs. In 770 cases of thalidomide damage arm was affected in 53.1%, arm + leg in 25.1%, arm + leg + ear in 1.9%, arm + ear in 5.7%, ear 11.2%, leg 1.2%, and internal organs only in 1.8%.

The causes of congenital failures are multiple. They may involve the implantation of the ovum and/or the formation or pathology of the placenta. Materno-em-bryonic nutritional imbalance may be a factor, e.g., copper or iron deficiency (+ other trace minerals?); deficiency of vitamins A, B, D, and certain endocrine imbalances, e.g., maternal thyroid malfunction or pancreatic malfunc-tion (diabetes).

Maternal diet is very important during pregnancy, not alone with reference to caloric intake, but also with refer-ence to protein, mineral, and vitamin.

This will be discussed in a later chapter.

In recent years *rubella* (German measles) has been revealed as a serious cause of congenital defects, ranging from organ defects to skeletal anomalies (among these are cleft palate and defective mineralization and linear growth of the long bones). The development of the measles vaccine has resulted in the acquisition of an immunity. Females who have had rubella, or are inoculated against it, have the antibodies necessary to counteract the rubella virus, so that it is no longer the threat that it was in the early months (first trimester) of pregnancy.

Radiation has been experimentally demonstrated as a definite cause, especially in the very early phases of cleavage and differentiation. As a general rule, after an exposure to X-rays, the cells most damaged are those scheduled to be most active *after* the moment (or time) of raying. For example in rats rayed at days 9–10–11 after conception there were eye and jaw defects (cleft palate and/or lip) and hydrocephaly (so-called "water on the brain"); rats rayed between 10–16 days showed skeletal defects in 485 of 622 young from 144 mothers.

The first trimester of pregnancy in humans is the particularly sensitive period. It is during this time that the physician-patient relationship should be maximally close in order that the entire maternal regime be as normal as possible, with reference to health, nutrition, therapeutic drug use, radiation, and so on.

The problem of spontaneous abortion or miscarriage is one of concern, for it occurs in about fifteen per cent of all pregnancies. A miscarriage may be somewhat arbitrarily defined as a uterine pregnancy terminated at six and one-half months or less. Large families are most frequently hit. There is no correlation with completeness of the family, maternal age, pregnancy spacing, or socioeconomic status. There are no significant ethnic differences. The risk of another abortion where there is a history of a previous abortion is about 25%; where there is no such history it is reduced to about 12%. If there is a defective child in the family the risk of abortion is 14.7%, which is almost identical with the 14.2% risk where all sibs are normal. In families with a pair of monozygotic twins (identical) or where there are sibs with cleft palate and/or cleft lip the risk is higher. It may be that maternal age, paternal age, and birth order are factors; if so, maternal age is the more important. In such cases it is likely that chromosomal aberrations are involved, rather than gene mutations. The risk that a given pregnancy will abort varies from woman to woman, and from year to year in the same woman.

The Newborn Child

In the normal, healthy newborn child there are a few interesting relationships to be noted—relation to maternal size, relation to birth order and so on. The correlation between maternal stature and fetal size is positive, but low. First-born babies tend to be smaller than later-born in dimensions of the head, trunk, and limbs; for weight, body length, and head circumference the differences are .18 kg, .34 cm, and .14 cm, respectively. The correlation between body size and birth order is positive but low. In postnatal growth, up to fourteen years, there is an inverse relationship between stature and birth order, i.e., first-borns average about one cm taller.

Birth-order has often been linked to mental ability or intellectual achievement. A California study suggested that *later* brothers and sisters in a family tended to have a slightly higher I.Q. On the other hand, a count in *Who's Who, American Men of Science,* and Rhodes scholars showed that first-borns were more frequent. In a 1953 study reporting on sixty-four "eminent scientists," it was said that seventy-two per cent were actually or effectively (were second-born but reared as first-born due to death of latter) the eldest son. In a series of 1618 high school students who were finalists in National Merit competition, sixty per cent who came from 2-3-4-5 children families were first-born. It does seem possible to conclude that ordinal position at birth is related to significant social parameters for reasons that at present are unknown or unclear.

There is a method of scoring the condition of the newborn, known as the *Apgar Score,* based on five clinical traits or assessments:

Score	Heart Rate	Respiratory Effect	Reflex Irritability	Muscle Tone	Color
2	100–140	Normal cry	Normal	Good	Pink
1	< 100	Irregular, shallow	Moderately depressed	Fair	Fair
0	No beat obtained	Apnea for 60 sec. + (transient cessation of breathing)	Absent	Flaccid	Cyanotic ("blue")

Determined within one minute after birth a score of 8–10 = good condition, 3–7 = fair, 0–2 = poor.

The Apgar Score is an attempt to evaluate the total well-being of the newborn child, yet only part of it can be objectified, while part of it is a more or less subjective clinical appraisal. Heart rate yields to tabulation via count, but the other four traits are related to the clinician's experience with variability: a "normal cry" is a good, lusty yell propelled from vigorous lungs; "reflex irritability" refers to elicited reflex responses, from marked ("normal") to absent; muscle tone is an appraisal of flexion-extension of limbs, turning of head, etc.; color can, of course, be reasonably well objectified, but "fair" is in mid pink-blue continuum. The scores, as totaled, give an acceptable prognosis of postnatal growth and development.

Culture and Child-Rearing

In contemporary American culture, young mothers are frequently confronted with two "problems," one fairly immediate, the other more or less emergent as the baby gets older. The first problem centers around the breast-bottle dichotomy, the second around the sleep-wakeful-ness rhythm. True information on these problems is es-sentially in the realms of hearsay and folklore. I know of only one truly longitudinal study of these problems, and it covers only the first three years of postnatal growth.

The problem of *breast-feeding* is a blend of manners and nutrition, so to speak. By "manners" is meant the sum-total of attitudes and cultural values. Certain it is, if we accept the data of anthropologists, that "primitive" peoples breast-feed the child not only more frequently, but for a much longer period of time. Swedish studies on contemporary urban populations show that boy babies breast-feed longer than girl babies. If the mother is over twenty-six years of age she is more apt to breast-feed for a longer time. Mothers in the higher socio-economic groups or who have had higher education breast-feed for a longer time. It is interesting that (in Sweden) mothers who live in "old-fashioned houses" stop breast-feeding earlier than those in up-to-date modern houses. In personality traits the mothers who breast-feed for six months or longer are more self-confident, secure, orderly, and calm.

The *sleep-patterns* in the first three years of life were noted by Swedish pediatricians. At age three years the child will sleep two and a half hours less per twenty-four hours than the child at six months. It is difficult to predict the length of sleep at any later growth-stage. In the first three years the incidence of night-waking is never less than twenty-three per cent; it is highest—seventy-five per cent—at one month. The tendency to wakefulness is a function of habituation to familial life-patterns; it is re-lated, for example, to over-crowding and/or prolonged breast-feeding.

III

GROWTH IN HEIGHT AND WEIGHT

The Problem of Size

How tall is tall? How short is short?

When is a child underweight? Overweight?

These are not simply rhetorical questions. The bounds of tallness and shortness, of under- and overweight, are in part problems of definition, and are certainly basic to the evaluation of satisfactory vs. unsatisfactory growth. In addition height and weight may be matters of great individual concern, for considerable cultural value is placed on size and body-build. There is a social premium upon the tall, athletically built male, and the moderately tall, slender, graceful female. Questions most frequently posed by parents (especially by the father) are, "How tall, how big, will my boy be?" or (by the mother), "Will my girl be too tall?" Whenever I am the target for these questions I begin to probe for motivation. Does *size* mean to the father that he possibly hopes to relive, in his boy, the athletic prowess that eluded him? Does *size* mean to the mother that she fears that a big girl will have more trouble finding a husband? Too often the concern of the parent(s) is arbitrarily imposed upon the child.

This business of being tall or short is seen by the size-prestige situations of adult life. In a recent Sunday newspaper supplement I came across the following: the Metropolitan Life Insurance Co. reports that average life insurance coverage is twice as much for six-footers as for five-footers; bishops average 5′10½″, rural preachers 5′8¾″; presidents of major Universities are 1″ taller than those of smaller colleges and of high school principals; sales managers hit 5′10″, their salesmen average 1″ shorter; railroad presidents are 5′11″, station agents 5′9½″; in the depression of the 1930's shorter men were first to be laid off; in fifteen Presidential elections victory went to the taller candidate (Lincoln was the tallest at 6′4″, LBJ next at 6′3″). And yet no one has ever *proved* that "bigger is better" or that "more is better." We Americans tend culturally to pay off on mere size and mass. In sports, particularly, each inch or each ten pounds is often worth more "on the hoof" at contract time.

I think that we Americans have made a cult, a fetish, out of the average. Ours is a culture of stereotypes, of rigid conformity. We set up "standards" and "norms" and then regard them as absolutes. If a boy or girl is "so old" he or she should be "so tall," or "weigh so much." Thus we set up height-for-age, weight-for-height categories and then expect an individual boy or girl to be at or near the average ("the great plateau of mediocrity," as it has been termed).

What has just been said does not deny for a moment that height and weight are the universally accepted criteria of normal, healthy physical growth; they are, carefully taken, precise, standardized yardsticks of growth progress. So long as the child is *fitted* into—not *forced* into—size categories of stature and weight there is no real objection. In this chapter I hope to make that clear.

There are several questions to answer as we evaluate a child's height-weight status and progress for age: 1) Is his or her *size* acceptable for age, sex, ethnic or national background, familial pattern, socio-economic group, and so on? 2) Is his or her *rate* acceptable for, say, the past year or two, or for a more extended period of time as, say, early or late childhood? 3) If the child has a growth problem (usually retarded growth), can a favorable *change in rate* be effected?

We can answer question 1) by reference to tables of normative data and by reference to a *distance curve* of growth, i.e., literally ascertain how far the child has traveled on the path toward maturity. Question 2) can be answered by noting *incremental* growth (the amount of gain in a given period of time—quarterly, semiannually, or annually) and by reference to a *velocity* curve which denotes speed of progress. Question 3) can be answered only in part; certainly, incremental growth can be noted, but a graphic growth curve here—an *acceleration* curve— is not yet developed.

Tables and Graphs of Height and Weight

In October 1959, the U.S. Public Health Service began a National Health Examination, in which samples of thousands of children are being studied in key geographic areas of the entire United States. The data from that survey are not yet available. We have data from purely local areas—Boston, Philadelphia, Cleveland, Yellow Springs, Iowa City, Denver, Berkeley—but no over-all data for U.S. children as a whole. In 1960, Stoudt, Damon, and McFarland reported to the Office of U.S. Surgeon General the results of a synthesis of all previously reported data on U.S. children. They came up with *pooled* height-weight-age data, from which Table I (p. 34) has been adapted: height in inches, weight in pounds, for boys and girls, birth to twenty-two years of age. For each dimension, for sex and age, the average or mean (M) and the standard deviation (S.D.) are given. The mean is literally a *central tendency* around which variability will cluster. The standard deviation is an expression of the *normal range of variation.* (See Appendix I.)

Look at a one-year-old baby boy, as an example: his length is 29.7″ with an S.D. of 1.1″; this means that sixty-

seven per cent of all one-year-old baby boys will be between 29.7″ + 1.1″ and 29.7″ − 1.1″, or 28.6″ and 30.8″;
similarly, 95 per cent will be between 29.7″ + 2 (1.1) or
29.7″ − 2 (1.1), or 27.5″−31.9″. Assume that we had a
one-year-old baby boy at M + 3 S.D. or 29.7″ + 3 (1.1″)
or 29.7″ + 3.3″ = 33″. This is really a long one-year-old
baby boy, at about the 99.2 per cent (at random only
eight in a thousand such male babies will be as long, or
longer). The point is, however, that statistically this is an
unusually long one-year-old boy—*not* an abnormally long
one!

What about the problem of weight, specifically of the
infant who is not "gaining weight" as he should? First of
all, it is probably more healthy to be a bit below in weight
than to be above. But if there is a slowing down in rate
of weight-gain so that the infant progressively goes to a
lower percentile, then there is cause for referring the baby
to the pediatrician. It is generally accepted that there are
three main causes for inadequate weight gain: 1) deficient
or defective intake in kind and/or amount of food
(breast-milk may be insufficient, or formula too dilute);
2) defective utilization by the digestive apparatus, probably due to biochemical imbalances; 3) defective utilization due to metabolic or systemic diseases. Weight loss
may occur in chronic diarrhea, ulcerative colitis and—
through excessive fluid loss—by overheating and over-
dressing.

In Figures 5–6 the data of Table I (p. 34) are plotted
for height and weight, respectively. These are *distance*
curves, with dimension plotted against time. In the height
curve it is to be noted that the girls' curve crosses the
boys' at 10:0, and for 11:0, 12:0, 13:0 the girls are, on the
average, taller than the boys. Similarly, the girls' weight
curve crosses the boys' at 11:0 and for 12:0 and 13:0 the
girls are, on the average, heavier than the boys.

Now a word about the variability of the height-weight
relationship. In Table I (p. 34) a 5:0 girl is 43.8″ (S.D.
1.7″) and 41.0 lbs. (S.D. 5.0 lbs.). Does this mean that a

32   *Child Growth*

GROWTH IN HEIGHT (INCHES)

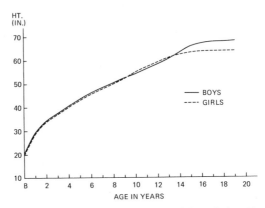

FIG. 5. Growth in Height, Birth to Adulthood (22 Years).

GROWTH IN WEIGHT (POUNDS)

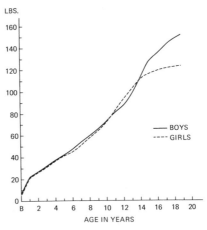

FIG. 6. Growth in Weight, Birth to Adulthood (22 Years).

43.8″ girl at 5:0 *must* weigh 41.0 lbs, and vice versa? Decidedly not! There are too many variable factors. Here is an example: in a Cleveland study twelve 5:0 girls, chosen at random from a total series of several hundred, averaged 42 lbs in weight, with a height range of 42.1″–45.5″

(3.4″). The weight of the girls at each quartile (each 25%) of the height range was 37 lbs, 40 lbs, 44 lbs and 47 lbs, respectively. The total weight range of these 12 girls was 30–63 lbs (33 lbs), which is 78.5 per cent of the mean weight for the sample!

In the earlier part of this chapter I asked several questions about height-weight data; one of them was about *size*—for age, for sex, for ethnic or national background, for familial pattern, for socio-economic group, and so on. Age and sex are covered in Table I. What about ethnic or national background? In time the American white traces back to Europe whence he or his ancestors emigrated. There are areas in Europe of tallness, and areas of shortness; for example, the peoples of northwestern and western Europe, especially the Scandinavians, are taller than the peoples of the circum-Mediterranean areas of southwestern and southeastern Europe; that is, northern Europeans *average taller*, southern Europeans *average* shorter. Practically this means that a boy of Swedish descent has a greater chance of being a +1 S.D. (above the mean), an Italian (from southern Italy, especially) a greater chance of being −1 S.D. (below the mean). This is, of course, random chance. Now, what about "familial pattern"? We will tackle this in greater detail in a later chapter on genetics, but right now we may generalize that tall parents are more likely to have tall children and short parents short children. If the father is 6′3″, mother 5′10″, and the 10:0 boy is at +2 S.D. for height the chances are that is where he belongs; but if he is at −2 S.D. for height then this signals the need for a careful scrutiny as to *why* he's so short when his genetic potential suggests otherwise. What about "socio-economic group"? Again, this will be taken up in a later chapter, but certainly the sum of all the circumstances—nutrition, health and health care, parent-child relationship, and so on—must be taken into consideration. There are intraurban, interurban, and urban-rural living conditions to be taken into consideration. The

TABLE I

HEIGHTS AND WEIGHTS OF AMERICAN CHILDREN

	MALES				FEMALES			
Age	Height (in.)		Weight (lbs.)		Height (in.)		Weight (lbs.)	
	M.	S.D.	M.	S.D.	M.	S.D.	M.	S.D.
Birth	20.0	1.0	7.6	1.3	19.7	1.0	7.5	1.1
3 mos.	23.5	1.0	13.0	1.8	23.05	1.0	12.0	1.4
6 "	26.3	1.0	17.4	2.05	25.05	1.0	16.3	1.85
9 "	28.15	1.1	20.55	2.35	27.5	1.0	19.0	2.15
1 yr.	29.7	1.1	23.0	3.0	29.3	1.0	21.6	3.0
2 yrs.	34.5	1.2	28.0	3.0	34.1	1.2	27.0	3.0
3 "	37.8	1.3	32.0	3.0	37.5	1.4	31.0	4.0
4 "	40.8	1.9	37.0	5.0	40.6	1.6	36.0	5.0
5 "	43.7	2.0	42.0	5.0	43.8	1.7	41.0	5.0
6 "	46.1	2.1	47.0	6.0	45.7	1.9	45.0	5.0
7 "	48.2	2.2	54.0	7.0	47.9	2.0	50.0	7.0
8 "	50.4	2.3	60.0	8.0	50.3	2.2	58.0	11.0
9 "	52.8	2.4	66.0	8.0	52.1	2.3	64.0	11.0
10 "	54.5	2.5	73.0	10.0	54.6	2.5	72.0	14.0
11 "	56.8	2.6	82.0	11.0	57.1	2.6	82.0	18.0
12 "	58.3	2.9	87.0	12.0	59.6	2.7	93.0	18.0
13 "	60.7	3.2	99.0	13.0	61.4	2.6	102.0	18.0
14 "	63.6	3.2	113.0	15.0	62.8	2.5	112.0	19.0
15 "	66.3	3.1	128.0	16.0	63.4	2.4	117.0	20.0
16 "	67.7	2.8	137.0	16.0	63.9	2.2	120.0	21.1
17 "	68.3	2.6	143.0	19.0	64.1	2.2	122.0	19.0
18 "	68.5	2.6	149.0	20.0	64.1	2.3	123.0	17.0
19 "	68.6	2.6	153.0	21.0	64.1	2.3	124.0	17.0
22 "	68.7	2.6	158.0	23.0	64.0	2.4	125.0	19.0

whole child in the *whole* environment is the focal point of evaluation.

Let us turn, now, to Table II (p. 37) and Figures 7–8, which deal with incremental growth and with velocity. Table II presents increments or amounts of height and weight growth between stated periods of time: thus a baby boy gains 3.5″ and 5.4 lbs in the first three postnatal months, a baby girl 3.35″ and 4.5 lbs, as calculated from Table I (again, these are averages).

In Figure 7 is plotted the velocity curve of height growth. There is a "peaking" of the curve in early child-

INCREMENTAL GROWTH IN HEIGHT (INCHES)

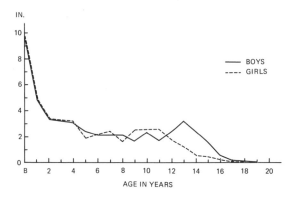

FIG. 7. Incremental Growth in Height, Birth to Adulthood (22 Years).

hood with height growth soaring to 4.8″ in both sexes in the 1–2 year period, and holding a mean annual gain of about 3″ through the 4–5 year period. The velocity then decelerates to about 8:0 in girls, about 11:0 in boys—then it accelerates (sweeps up) for two-three years in girls, two-four years in boys. This upsweep, which is, on the average, two years *earlier in girls* is called by some "the adolescent spurt," by others the "prepubertal accelera- tion" or "circumpubertal acceleration." At all events, this is when the boy or girl "shoots up" in height, or "grows like a weed." Figure 7 emphasizes female priority in height growth: girls are about two years ahead of boys.

In Figure 8 is plotted the velocity curve of weight growth. Here the curve for both sexes sweeps up and to the right, a gradually increasing velocity. The weight "spurt" is ten to fourteen years in girls, twelve to fifteen years in boys, with the girls once more showing a two- year precocity, compared to boys. Note the far greater velocity in boys. The weight gain in girls has a high sub-

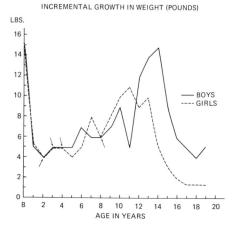

FIG. 8. Incremental Growth in Weight, Birth to Adulthood (22 Years).

cutaneous fat layer component, in boys a muscle-bone component.

For normal healthy children, age 5½–17½ years, Massler and Suher of Chicago have provided formulae for the prediction of "normal" or "ideal" weight in children. The formulae are based on but two simple measurements: height and calf circumference, both in cm, to give weight in gms.

$$\text{Boys} \quad \frac{(calf\ circ.)^2}{3.247} \times H = W$$
$$\text{Girls} \quad \frac{(calf\ circ.)^2}{3.334} \times H = W$$

$H = \text{height}$

$W = \text{weight}$

The correlation between actual and predicted weight is extremely high: boys = +.9902, girls = +.99994. This is almost perfect correlation.

We Are Growing Bigger

A fact to be observed is that height-weight tables more than twenty-five years old are outdated, for American boys and girls are taller and heavier today than their brothers

TABLE II

INCREMENTAL GROWTH IN HEIGHT AND WEIGHT
OF AMERICAN WHITE CHILDREN

Age	MALES Height (in.)	Weight (lbs.)	FEMALES Height (in.)	Weight (lbs.)
B–3 mos.	3.5	5.4	3.35	4.5
3–6 "	2.8	4.4	2.0	4.3
6–9 "	1.85	3.15	2.45	2.7
9 mos.–1 yr.	1.55	2.45	1.8	2.6
1–2 yrs.	4.8	5.0	4.8	5.4
2–3 "	3.3	4.0	3.4	4.0
3–4 "	3.0	5.0	3.1	5.0
4–5 "	2.9	5.0	3.2	5.0
5–6 "	2.4	5.0	1.9	4.0
6–7 "	2.1	7.0	2.2	5.0
7–8 "	2.2	6.0	2.4	8.0
8–9 "	2.4	6.0	1.8	6.0
9–10 "	1.7	7.0	2.5	8.0
10–11 "	2.3	9.0	2.5	10.0
11–12 "	1.5	5.0	2.5	11.0
12–13 "	2.4	12.0	1.8	9.0
13–14 "	2.9	14.0	1.4	10.0
14–15 "	2.7	15.0	0.6	5.0
15–16 "	1.4	9.0	0.5	3.0
16–17 "	0.6	6.0	0.2	2.0
17–18 "	0.2	6.0	0.0	1.0
18–19 "	0.1	4.0	0.0	1.0
19–22 "	0.1	5.0	—0.1	1.0

and sisters of yesterday. This phenomenon is called "the secular increase in size." To a greater or less degree it is characteristic of all peoples who share in the cultural advances of present-day Western or Occidental civilization.

Meredith of Iowa has surveyed this secular trend to taller and heavier American children, reporting for boys on data covering the period 1880–1960. In Figure 9 are presented the height distance curves for 1880–1960 and in Figure 10 the weight distance curves for 1880–1960 (American white boys).

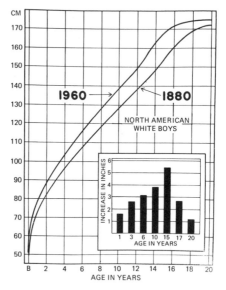

FIG. 9. Secular Trend in Height, 1880–1960.

American Negro children are also showing a secular trend to height-weight growth, but less markedly so.

Why are Americans becoming taller and heavier? Many reasons have been given and I have organized these reasons in major categories as follows:

I. Health and nutrition

    1. Decline in frequency of growth-retarding illness, especially in the first five years of life.

    2. Improvement of amount and balance of nutritional intake, including vitamin supplementation; a corollary here may be a reduction in family size in the middle-class brackets, so that total available food supply is spread over a smaller total family unit.

    3. Improvement in medical care and personal health practices.

4. Improvement in living (housing) conditions and over-all community hygiene, i.e., the availability of community health services.

There is no doubt that these four factors are basic to the facilitation of optimum growth of the child. If the normal child achieves about one half his adult stature by two years, then any debilitating illness in this period must

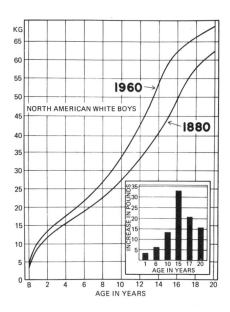

FIG. 10. Secular Trend in Weight, 1880–1960.

be inhibitory to a marked degree. Remove the illness and its causes and the period of normal rapid growth proceeds unchecked. Add a good all-around diet and the effects of good health are compounded. In this cultural improvement shared alike by the individual and by his total milieu then health and nutrition go hand-in-hand with good growth.

II. Socio-economic conditions

1. Reduction in child labor
2. Reversal of a biological adaptation to hard labor and crowded living conditions.

These two factors are mentioned most often in the studies of child growth in the British Isles. In the nineteenth century child labor in coal mines and the big mills exacted a repressive toll upon the health and stamina of the growing child. Work conditions were often wretched to an unbelievable degree. Additionally, the crowding within and around industrial centers made for wretched slum living conditions. Child labor in England and Scotland, as in the United States, has been greatly reduced, so that children are freed to grow under far less repressive circumstances. Slums—urban "ghettos"—are still with us and still impact their own measures of inhibited growth.

III. Genetic factors

1. Cumulative expression of hybrid vigor
2. Changes in the U.S. population due to immigration
3. Assortative mating.

It is a well-established fact in biology that interbreeding results in *heterosis* or hybrid vigor, in that the crossing-products in the first few generations are bigger (in size, in weight, or both). In America, the "melting pot," there are so many ethnic intermarriages that the resulting offspring benefit by this heterotic effect. Another suggestion is that those who emigrate to the United States from Europe are often the tallest, strongest, and boldest. Finally, on a like-calls-to-like basis, it is suggested that the taller males and females of each generation marry to perpetuate the gained tallness.

The possible genetic effects of population intermixtures

are worth considering, but they are subordinate to the factors of I and II, above.

IV. Individual-personal improvement

    1. Increase in exercise and athletic participation
    2. Change to less restrictive and lighter clothing.

There is no convincing evidence that either of these factors has played a significant role in the secular trend to larger size.

v. Evolutionary trend

    1. Tendency for members of a major evolutionary group to increase progressively in size.

In the paleontological record this tendency can be seen in many animals, such as dinosaurs, titanotheres, the elephant, the horse, and so on. But in my opinion this kind of an explanation does not fit man, in the sense of the great recency of human size increase.

I am often asked, "When will this size-increase business stop?" My answer is twofold: 1) the fossil evidence shows that early humans were variable in size; their long bones show calculated statures ranging from short to moderately tall. My feeling is that man has always had a potential for tallness—now, for the first time, it is being realized because inhibitory factors have been greatly lessened; 2) the curve of height-increase is already leveling off in the last generation or so.

Are we going to be a race of giants? I answer, No! Man may achieve an average of 6′ or so for males, 5′6″ or so for females, but that is, and will be, his species boundary.

There is a secular trend in foot length, also, but I hasten to add that our feet are getting only relatively bigger—we have bigger feet because we're a taller people. Today the shoe-size of the average American white male is 9–10 B, but "Gran'pa" averaged size 7A–B, a 2–3 size gain.

American male feet have grown ⅓″ longer per generation. The ladies share in this: today one of six American women wears a size 9 shoe or larger. [This is quite an item, economically speaking: about 650 million pairs of shoes are sold annually; add ⅓″ of leather needed per generation and you get about 6,800 miles of additional shoe leather—diagonally from Maine to California.]

The ratio of foot length to stature (foot L/Ht.) has not changed, for we are getting proportionately larger. If fourteen-year-old Jim has a shoe-size equal to Dad's, or thirteen-year-old Margie one equal to Mom's, it is only because Jim and Margie may be absolutely taller as adults, and they'll be relatively taller as teen-agers. The size factor may well be one aspect of "the generation gap"!

The Prediction of Adult Height

Can adult stature and weight be predicted? Here is a "rule of thumb":

Boys: 2 × height at age 2 = adult height; 5 × weight at age 2 = adult weight.

Girls: 2 × height at 1½ years = adult height; 5 × weight at 1½ years = adult weight.

"Rules" such as this probably apply only to children who, at a given age up to 2:0, are within a normal range of variation (M ± 1 S.D., or two of three children). Later on, chronological age must defer to biological or maturational age. An *early maturing* child will probably be shorter as an adult than predicted from stature as a child. Conversely, a *late-maturing* child will probably be taller as an adult than predicted from stature as a child. If we go back to birth size, prediction is even less accurate. Birth weight and adult weight are positively correlated, +0.35, but low; similarly birth length and adult height show a low correlation, +0.30.

In 1952 Bayley and Pinneau of Berkeley, California, published tables for the estimation of adult stature. These tables were based on the relation of chronological age to biologic or maturation age (the latter determined by the assessment of the stage of development of the bones of hand and wrist as seen in an X-ray film). Three developmental categories were set up: 1) *average,* when the maturation age was within ± one year of the chronological age; 2) *accelerated,* when the maturation age was more than one year advanced over the chronological age; 3) *retarded,* when the maturation age was more than one year behind the chronological age. Let me use a ten-year-old boy as an example (the same example applies to a girl):

1) chronological age = ten years
   maturation age   = between nine and eleven years
   this is an *average* boy, for his maturation age is within one year (±) of his chronological age
2) chronological age = ten years
   maturation age   = eleven years, six months
   this is an *accelerated* boy, for his maturation age is 1½ years beyond his chronological age
3) chronological age = ten years
   maturation age   = eight years, six months
   this is a *retarded* boy, for his maturation age is 1½ years behind his chronological age

The chronological age, the maturation age, and the actual stature at age ten are then referred to appropriate tables (Average, Accelerated, Retarded) for the boy or for the girl as the case may be. I have used these tables for many years and found them quite reliable in prediction.

I have chosen to illustrate the use of the tables by a case history of a California boy followed for twenty-one years by Bayer and Bayley (1959); the case is graphed in Figure 11 (p. 44). The top set of distance curves, sloping up from left to right are as follows: the lower dashed curve is a retarded case; the mid three lines are the average, minus one standard deviation (below) and plus one standard deviation (above); the heavy line is the boy's

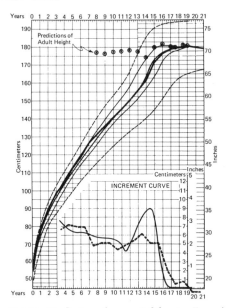

FIG. 11. Height Prediction for a California Boy (see text for details).

actual height curve; he follows the average closely; the top dashed line is an accelerated case. The bottom two curves plot the annual increments in height (solid line) and in weight (barred line). The "hump," in the height incremental curve represents the "adolescent height spurt."

The important information in Figure 11 is at the very top of the graph. Between eight and nineteen years of age there were thirteen annual height predictions (of adult height): they all cluster between 175–185 cm; actually he was 180 cm at age nineteen.

What about the growing girl who is "too tall"? Obviously the definition of "too tall" is subjective and is related to familial and ethnic size. A girl 5' 7" with parents of 6' or more will not stand out as does a 5' 7" girl with parents well under 6'. Similarly, a girl of Scandinavian parents will be taller, as a rule, than a girl of South Italian parents. The problem of "too tall" is usually set by parental concern: parents feel that over 76″ for boys and over 70″ for girls represent an upper limit, beyond which personal and psycho-social discomfort may be felt.

The girl can be "stopped" from growing taller, but such a procedure should be attempted only under the care of a physician who is a specialist in endocrinology. The inhibition of height growth may be effected by the administration of the female sex hormone (estrogen, usually in the form of stilbestrol). This hormone accelerates the union of the growing ends of the long bones with the main portion or shaft; as a result the long bones (of the legs in the case of stature) no longer grow (no longer increase in length).

In an Australian study of sixteen girls whose predicted adult height, estimated at 13½ years, was 179.3 cm (70.6″) the actual attained stature was 175.2 cm (68.9″); treatment duration was 19½ months during which time three milligrams of stilbestrol were given daily. Age of beginning treatment is very important. In the study of these sixteen girls six were treated *before* first menstruation and in them adult stature was 6.4 cm less than predicted; five girls were treated within twelve months *after* first menstruation, and their adult stature was only 3.6 cm less than predicted; five girls were treated a year or more *after* first menstruation and their adult stature was only 1.8 cm less than predicted.

Is there a *seasonal* effect on growth? I am not going to answer this more than to say that a number of studies suggest *height* gain in spring-summer, *weight* gain in fall-winter. This may be only in part "seasonal" in terms of more sun, less sun, more rain, less rain, hot vs. cold, and so on. There are cultural factors, in that weight gain may be a reflection of reduced exercise, increased sedentary life, in the colder months.

The Obese Child

Obesity in children is a vexing problem. In the first place obesity has never been properly defined. It seems to be a subjective thing: it is what others think it is, i.e., people look at a heavy child and say, "he or she is obese" (usually a "she" is referred to).

The U.S. Public Health Service stated that obesity probably has an hereditary basis—at least it tends to run in families: seventy-five per cent of children called "too fat" had at least one very overweight (obese) parent; children of overweight parents have a ninety per cent chance of being themselves obese.

In principle a very careful study of Seltzer and Mayer (1964) of Harvard confirms that a tendency to obesity in girls has a genetic basis, related essentially to a heritable body-build pattern. They studied a sample of one hundred and eighty healthy white American obese adolescent girls (age-range 11.6–18 yrs., mean 15.04 yrs., with ninety-five percent between twelve and seventeen years). They were from all over the U.S., but seventy-six per cent were from the northeast; ninety-five per cent were of native-born, middle- or upper-class parents; forty per cent were Jewish, sixty per cent stemmed from northwestern and western Europe. Certain body dimensions plus skinfold thicknesses were measured.

The one hundred-eighty girls were "persistent obesities of long standing." Their average weight was 170¾ lbs (77.4 kgs). As a group they were forty-six per cent overweight on the 1959 Berkeley standards of Bayer and Bayley; ninety-three per cent of the sample was 20+ per cent overweight; seventy-three per cent of the sample was 30+ per cent overweight; thirty-five per cent of the sample was 50+ per cent overweight.

In general the deposition of fat in the obese child is largely just below the skin, and is measured by skincalipers. A fold of skin is picked up between thumb and forefinger and is measured by the calipers that have a carefully controlled spring tension. There are two skinfolds that most accurately measure subcutaneous fat: 1) *tricipital,* at mid-level on the back of the left upper arm; 2) *subscapular,* on the back just below the lowest part of the left shoulder blade. A thickness of more than 20 mm (⅘″) for each skinfold was arbitrarily set as the lower limit of obesity. In the one hundred and eighty girls the average tricipital skinfold was 38 mm; for the subscapular skinfold the average was 33 mm. These two averages of 38 mm and 33 mm were, respectively, two and three times *greater* than for a control non-obese group.

Certain body breadth measurements were taken, based on bony structures definitely *not* the sites of subcutaneous fat deposition. These were as follows: shoulder breadth, elbow breadth, wrist breadth, hand breadth ("across the knuckles") and ankle breadth. In all of these bony or skeletal breadths the girls classed as "obese" were significantly larger, i.e., they had a more "robust" skeletal framework.

There is another fact of import, namely, that the excessively fat girls grow faster—a greater growth velocity —and mature earlier.

Seltzer and Mayer conclude that "the greater skeletal dimensions of our obese adolescent girls seems to reflect inherent differences in bodily structure, over and beyond what might be attributed to the effects of accelerated development or of long-term overnourishment."

It must be pointed out that body-build almost certainly is only one aspect of the total problem, basic though morphology may be. Endocrine and psychological factors must be considered and evaluated. The obese boy or girl must receive adequate medical, nutritional, and psychologic (psychiatric) counseling.

Concluding Remarks

Some forty years ago, when I first began to study child growth, the prevailing tendency was to demand that the child walk the straight and narrow path of the average: average height, average weight, average weight-for-height. I am reminded of a cartoon I saw a few years ago in the *New Yorker:* a physician was depicted examining a very portly gentleman, and the caption read, "Sir, for your weight you should be 11′ 8¼″ tall!" This cartoon is not much sillier than literally "pouring" a child into an arbitrary H-W container.

Today we regard the path of individual growth progress as more of a broad highway along which the child may saunter; now veering a bit to one side (height gain) now a bit to the other (weight gain) but in good health always keeping his inherited and constitutional growth-form in balance. He'll be, as he grows, taller or shorter, lighter or heavier than the average.

But there's a joker here. When are taller or shorter, lighter or heavier, significant, i.e., when are they cause for concern in the sense of *too* tall, *too* short, *too* light (underweight), *too* heavy (overweight)?

To begin with, the section on *The Obese Child* gave data on girls only. There are obese boys, of course, but data on them are sparse. There are, I think, two reasons for this: 1) there are not so many obese boys as there are obese girls; and 2) parents are more concerned with obese girls (and the girl reacts accordingly) than they are with obese boys.

Now to the question: at what point, in terms of height and weight data, should there be an evaluation that John or Mary is significantly above or below the average (the fiftieth percentile)? Because there are a host of factors to be considered—familial patterns, ethnic background, and so on—I hesitate to give a hard-and-fast rule. Nevertheless, I venture that tenth percentile or below for height is very short, tenth percentile or below for weight is underweight; similarly, ninetieth percentile or above for height is very tall, ninetieth percentile or above for weight is overweight.

IV

BIOLOGICAL AGE: GROWTH AGE

Which Age?

In many respects this is a difficult chapter to write, for I
want to present a very important concept in the analysis
of child growth. When I was a lad, growing very fast, it
was said of me that "he is very tall for his age." I was
deemed tall on two counts: 1) comparison with age and
sex peers; and 2) compared to age-tables of stature. The
age-tables were, of course, based on the calendar, i.e.,
they were related to my birthday age. It was not until
some eighteen years later, when I was a graduate student,
that I learned I had several ages: I was, for example, as
old as my teeth in my childhood years; in these years I
was also as old as my bones. In other words I had an
inborn biologic age related to growth events and growth
timing; I learned that there were synonyms for this biological time-clock within my growing body: "maturation
age," "bone age," and "skeletal age." It is this latter term,
abbreviated to S.A., that I shall use in this chapter, for
the development of skeletal units is the tell-tale of how
really old the child is.

Assume that three American boys—either white or
Negro—are standing before you. Each is a healthy, adequately nourished ten-year-old boy. They were all born,
let us say, on July 1, 1961; hence, on July 1, 1971, each
boy, of either group, was ten years old by the calendar.

This is *chronological age* (C.A.). Most of our growth data, especially our measurement data (as for height, weight, and all linear dimensions) are based on C.A. When we say, "Johnny (or Mary) is ten years old" we mean, 999 times out of 1,000, that he or she is ten years old according to his or her birth date.

Now suppose I tell you that boy #1 is, in biological or maturational growth terms, only 8:6 (eight years, six months), boy #2 is indeed 10:0, while boy #3 is 11:6. With respect to C.A. boy #1 is *retarded* 1:6, boy #3 is *advanced* 1:6, and boy #2 is right on schedule. Instead of the identity of C.A. there is the disparity of developmental or growth age: there is a three year difference in biological age—or in growth-time—between boys #1 and #3. In other words boy #3 has a significantly greater maturational age than has boy #1.

The concept of "maturation age" is a basic one in the understanding of the *timing* and *rate* of child-growth. The postnatal growth period of twenty years is like a race: we all run it, but some run it fast, some slow. As a result, at some time during the twenty years, some children are ahead of others, some are behind. The ones who are "ahead" are biologically older; the ones who are "behind" are biologically younger. There is nothing startling about all this for it is just another way of saying that not all children grow alike.

Then why say it?

There are at least three good reasons why the child's biological growth-age should be considered: 1) it grants him his *right to individuality,* for biological growth is *his own,* and not an average; 2) it is a better measure of behavioral expectancy than is chronological age, i.e., a child functions and behaves more in accordance with his own innate age than his chronological age; 3) it is genetically entrenched, for growth "lateness" or "earliness" tends to run in family-lines.

The real question is this: "How is this biological growth-age, this maturation, measured?" Certainly the whole body matures—all systems, all organs, and so on. Which system shall we select as our basis of judgment?

The X-ray of the Skeleton

There is one system of the body that most readily tells the story of growth timing and growth rate, that tells us *how old the child* really is. This system involves the bones of the body, the entire skeleton. Bones can be clearly and easily seen via the X-ray film.

This is not the place to go into a long story about the growing skeleton. I shall give but one example, the tibia or shinbone, a long bone of the lower leg. It grows (or "ossifies") from three main centers, of which the mid or shaft is the largest; at each end are separate centers; the shaft is called the *diaphysis,* each end is called an *epiphysis.* Shaft and its ends are at first separated by cartilage and it is in this area where most of the growth occurs. Sometime in the late teens the cartilage becomes bone and the shaft "unites" with each end. Growth in length ceases, and the bone is said to be "adult."

We can take advantage of this bone growth and maturation picture by studying the X-ray of the hand, including the wrist. In this X-ray film there are no less than *fifty-one separate centers* of bone growth and maturation. In Figure 12 a hand-wrist X-ray film illustrates this.

Why the hand-wrist? There are several reasons. Pragmatically the hand is the most easily accessible part of the skeleton. Basically the end-points of observation (the *appearance* of a given center of bone growth, and its *union*—in all but the carpals) are clearly defined. The process of maturation is a continuous process that may be followed via serial X-ray films. Finally, the total process of assessing the bone-age, or skeletal age, is well standardized. We have *atlases* of hand maturation that are readily used. With some practice a hand-wrist X-ray film can be reliably "assessed"; the correlations within a single assessor, doing the films repeatedly over a period of time, and between assessors, is acceptably high.

Where do we draw the bounds of "early" or "advanced" and "late" or "retarded" S.A. with reference to

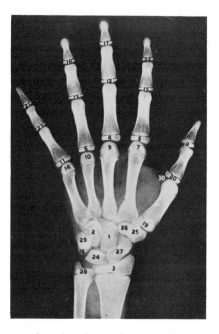

FIG. 12. X-ray Film of Left Hand-Wrist, Showing the Growing Bones.

C.A.? The hand X-ray film of a normal, healthy, six-year-old child was sent to forty-nine professional medical radiologists and each was asked to establish his own bounds of acceptability: eight said ±0:6 (5:6–6:6), twenty-one said ±1:0 (5:0–7:0); eight said ±1:6 (4:6–7:6); the other twelve had varying combinations. Those of us who work in the growth field now use the bounds of "normal" variation as C.A. ± 1:0 S.A., but we use judgment in this. For example, it is much more significant, possibly calling for a closer evaluation, when a child of 3:0 lags a year or more than when a child 12:0 correspondingly lags: in the 3:0 child the lag is thirty-three per cent, in the 12:0 child the lag is only eight per cent. In Figure 13 is an illustration of percentage groupings for Cleveland boys and girls, in terms of advanced, average, and retarded.*

PERCENTAGE GROUPINGS

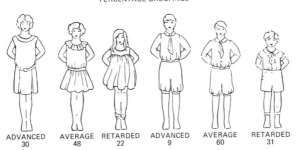

| ADVANCED | AVERAGE | RETARDED | ADVANCED | AVERAGE | RETARDED |
| 30 | 48 | 22 | 9 | 60 | 31 |

FIG. 13. Percentages of Advanced, Average, Retarded Skeletal Age in Cleveland Children.

Advanced or fast-growing children are more apt to be taller and heavier, retarded or slow-growing children are more apt to be shorter and lighter. Because maturation age is so firmly entrenched in the human child, as the basic register of growth-time, it is closely related to many other biological aspects of growth. In the pages that follow I shall enumerate and discuss the relation between S.A. and many other variables, most of them biological, a few cultural: sex differences; racial or ethnic differences including the cultural milieu; illness; nutrition; mental retardation; seasonal factors; genetic and familial background. There is a vast literature on all these variables but we must content ourselves with a paragraph or two on each.

*This is a forty-year-old drawing. Note that the boys are wearing knee pants. They have not yet "matured" enough to have earned "long pants." The girls are properly mini-skirted.

Brief Evaluation of Bio-Cultural Variables in Maturation

There is no doubt of a *sex* difference in maturation, with females advanced compared with males, a priority present at birth and continuing, at a rather constantly accelerated rate, until puberty, at the end of which time the boys catch up. As can be seen in Figure 14, there are "early" and "late" boys and girls, but in each category the girls are about two to three years ahead of the boys.

Skeletal development is also correlated with *puberty* (menarche, or onset of menstruation) in girls. In Cleveland children there was studied the onset of ossification in a forearm bone, in a small bone of the thumb, and in

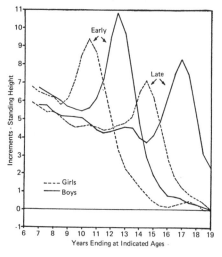

FIG. 14. Early and Late Maturing Boys and Girls.

the iliac crest of the pelvis. The correlation, respectively, with menarche was +0.62, +0.71, and +0.81. The ossification center for iliac crest appeared six months *before* menarche. It is likely that iliac crest onset in the boy triggers analogous pubertal changes with specific reference to changes in endocrine balance and/or dominance.

Whether or not there is a *racial* or *ethnic* difference in maturation is a question. If there is a real racial difference then it must be genetically entrenched. But this is difficult to demonstrate. Again, the problem of multiple factors has to be considered. In the United States there seems to be a real racial difference in favor of the American Negro infant, who is born with a more advanced bone development, compared to American white babies. This advantage—if it is an advantage—is held until three years of age; at this time the difference disappears, and from then on there are virtually identical age relationships and progress in skeletal maturation in white and Negro children.

We may accept as a general principle that skeletal maturation is relatively resistant to adverse *socio-economic* circumstances. Weight and height growth, in that order, will be inhibited or deviated long before the maturation is affected.

How the usual childhood *illnesses* affect S.A. is not clear. The appearance of a bone center may be delayed, but it will catch-up after a while. In Ohio children, for example, the ossification order or sequence did not, in a sample of one hundred and fifty-four children from birth to seven years, correspond with greater or fewer illness episodes (measles, chicken pox, mumps, "colds," and so on).

There can be no doubt that *nutrition* plays an important role in the entire bone-age process. In a 1963 study in Turkey one hundred eighty cases of malnutrition in babies from birth to 2:0 were divided into four degrees of malnutrition, in increasing order of severity: in the first degree nutritional group the children averaged eighty-nine per cent of the S.A. norm for age; in the second degree group the average was seventy-one per cent; in the third degree group the average was fifty-four per cent; and in the fourth degree group the average was forty per cent.

Illness and poor nutrition may leave their imprint in the skeleton. In the growing long bones are often to be seen, on the X-ray film, *lines and bands of increased density* (which show up whiter on the film). They are called "lines of arrested growth," for they are seen at the growing ends of the shaft of the long bone, or "transverse lines," since they are at right angles to the long axis of the shaft. Not only illness or malnutrition produce these transverse lines. They are frequently seen after blood transfusions in chronic or acute anemia, and also in children dwarfed because of hypopituitarism (failure of the growth hormone) who are receiving male hormone (testosterone) to aid in statural recovery. They are also seen in lead and phosphorus poisoning, and occasionally where too much vitamin D has been given. On occasion there is a "birth-line" or "neonatal" line which registers the trauma of birth.

The lines, once they have appeared, stay for a long time. Their position is so fixed that they may be used as "markers" from which to measure amount and rate of long-bone growth.

Mentally retarded children are often also retarded in skeletal maturation. In a Wisconsin study of thirty-eight boys (average age first seen 7:0–12:0) and twenty-six girls (average age first seen 7:0–11:0) who had Downs Syndrome ("mongolism"), and who were followed for four years, the average S.A. retardation was three years between 7:0–9:0, but at age 12:0 the retardation was only one year. It is quite likely that the skeletal retardation is not caused by the mental retardation per se, but is merely one aspect of the total set of factors that were initially causally related to the overall bio-behavioral deviation.

There may be a *seasonal* variation in skeletal maturation. In one study of one hundred thirty-three children, age 1:0–5:0, studied longitudinally, height, weight, and

S.A. were analyzed. In this particular study weight gain was most from October to December, least, from April to June. Height gain was most April to June, least October to December. Appearance of centers was most March to May, least September to November. Weight and height just reversed their most-least timing. The gain in S.A. was most-least at about the same times as for height gain. In this correlated study the seasonal variation seemed to be greatest in weight, next in maturation, and least in height.

Patterns of skeletal maturation are *genetically* governed. The evidence is not clear-cut: 1) it is difficult to define a specific aspect of the process as a unit; 2) there is no simple dominance or recessiveness; 3) data on human subjects are scant and incomplete. Nevertheless it seems reasonable to state that pattern of bone-growth is under more or less well-defined genetic control. In an Ohio study which included six pairs of identical twins, twenty-two pairs of brothers and sisters, eight pairs of first cousins, and nine pairs of non-relates, for all of whom longitudinal data were available, it was concluded that the maturation pattern was similar in the order of twins, siblings, cousins, and non-relates. A study of monozygote triplets (from a single fertilized egg) showed, over an 8:0–18:0 period, progressive changes in rate of skeletal maturation so that the rank-order of onset of bone development was different at different ages. It must be assumed that variable environmental factors, or acquired metabolic characteristics, are capable of modifying a genetic pattern of maturation.

Here are some twin data from the Philadelphia *Growth Center:*

	Pair #1			Pair #2	
	RK	LK		JMC	KMC
CA	(S.A.)	(S.A.)	C.A.	(S.A.)	(S.A.)
10:0	8.4	8:4	12:4	12:9	12:6
10:6	8:7	8:7	12:10	13:0	12:9
12:2	11:0	11:0	14:8	15:0	14:9

Pair #1 is uniformly and identically *retarded* in S.A.; both are *late maturers*.

Pair #2 are both slightly advanced, but not significantly so; J is a bit ahead of K.

The assessment of the maturation age of the child is far more than mere academic interest. It is true that we are culturally geared to the calendar and that we think of, and react to, a child in terms of birthday-years. Indeed, the data in books on child growth are to a great extent in terms of average chronological age. I hold a brief for maturation age, the real growing-older age of the child. I believe that this is the age that should provide the basic yardstick for the evaluation of the emergence of patterns of behavior—*including* learning behavior. Biological growth-time is innate; the child is born with it; he has inherited it; it is a basic factor in how he reacts to most of the cultural stimuli to which he is or will be exposed. I do not minimize the environment, for I know its potent impact. However, in the last analysis, the environment differs in its impact upon the maturationally advanced as compared to the maturationally retarded child. The former has, I feel, greater adaptability because of greater maturation.

V

GROWTH OF TRUNK, ARM, AND
LEG COMPONENTS AND OF
JAWS AND TEETH

The Rest of the Body

As one observes the growing child one notes that he is "getting bigger," and this observation usually is in terms of size—how *tall*—and weight—how *heavy*. The casual observer rarely goes beyond these two easily seen and objective phenomena of growth. This is not enough, by far. A ten-year-old child, or an adult, is not simply an infant "grown bigger"! He is a ten-year-old or an adult who has increased in size, changed in proportions, and increased in complexity of function in a certain way. There has been a veritable metamorphosis in the first ten years, the second ten years, and over the total twenty-year growth span.

In this chapter we must go beyond height and weight and find out how that height and that weight are made up. In the pages ahead I shall discuss how the trunk grows, how arm and leg grow, how face, jaws, and teeth grow. This can be done fairly easily by measurements of external form, but these measurements are not enough, for they do not give insight into how the trunk, the limbs, the head, are put together in terms of what may be called the "composition" or the "compartments" of the body.

I have tried in this book not to belabor the reader with too much tabulated material, but in this chapter I cannot escape a few lists of data or a few tables of measurements. After all a dimension or a ratio is an objective fact that literally speaks for itself; not only that, but a tabular con-centration, so to speak, is in the interests of efficiency—it says a lot in a limited space. This will be seen with special clarity when we look at body compartments and at the eruption of the teeth.

It is misleading to speak of height and weight as mea-sures of growth and to speak of them as though they were discrete units, the former linear, the latter volumetric. Height, from head to foot, is one straight over-all linear dimension. As such it seems quite simple; yet it involves many areas or structures of the whole body: head, neck, trunk, and arm and leg, and their segmental parts. Weight likewise seems to be a simple measure of mass; yet it is three-dimensional, at least: vertical, or top to bottom, transverse, or side to side, and sagittal, or front to back.

The child does not grow "all of a piece"; he grows, as has been earlier stated, differentially in all of his parts and systems. He changes sizes, he changes proportions, he changes times and rates of growth. There are so many such variables that it is *impossible to define an average child* in terms of any but one thing at a time. Here is an example of what I mean, based upon adult males (for whom growth-time was no longer a factor): in a sample of 4,063 men, *for only 10 measurements,* 1,055 (25.9%) were average in one measurement, 302 (7.4%) of these 1,055 were average in two measurements, 143 (3.5%) of the 302 in three, 73 (1.8%) of the 143 in four, 28 (0.69%) of the 73 in five, 12 (0.29%) of the 28 in six, six (0.14%) of the 12 in seven, three (0.07%) of the six in eight, two (0.04%) of the three in nine, and *none* of the last two in ten! It goes without saying that as the number of vari-ables (dimensions, proportions, structures, etc.) increases the sample size must become almost infinite. The best that we can ever do is to say that the whole growing child—for age, for sex, for race—is acceptable "somewhere within a normal range of variation." Growth is dynamic. In the healthy child it never stands still. Fortunately there is an order in the process, for the unfolding structural and functional pattern obeys time and sequence rules.

Figure 15 shows how stature is put together, from the second embryonic month to age 17 years, at which time stature is about ninety-five per cent of its adult value. The changing linear contributions to stature by head + neck, trunk, and leg show a regular sequence of interrelationship: head + neck shows a regular decrease, leg a regular increase, with trunk literally in between. This, then, demonstrates that stature is *not* a single linear measurement; instead it is a composite.

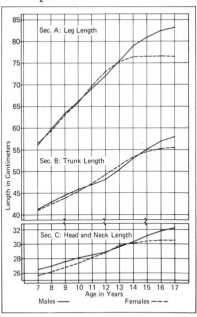

FIG. 15. Age-Changes in Contribution of Head and Neck, Trunk, and Leg to Stature.

Components of the Body

In a breakdown that may be overly simple, it is possible to say that there are five major structural components of the human body: 1) skin + superficial fat; 2) viscera, heart included; 3) the central and peripheral nervous system; 4) muscle; 5) bone. Here, too, there is a regular sequential change, from fetus to adult:

| | PER CENT OF TOTAL | | |
Structure	Fetus	Newborn	Adult
Skin + fat	16%	26%	25%
Viscera	16%	16%	11%
Nervous	21%	15%	3%
Muscle	25%	25%	43%
Skeleton	22%	18%	18%

The structural transition from birth to adulthood is quite regular for skin + fat, skeleton, and viscera. It shows a tremendous decrease in relative nervous system, and a corresponding increase in relative muscle mass.

Body composition of the newborn child may be expressed in a slightly different fashion, in what is termed "the male reference infant," who is made up something like this:

Structure	Weight in gms	Per cent of total weight
Body weight	3500 gms	—
Water	2628 gms	75%
Fat	385 gms	11%
Protein	399 gms	11.4%
Mineral	59 gms	1.7%
"Residue"	29 gms	0.8%
Fat-free body mass	3115 gms	89%

Now, on a percentage basis, let us note how this male reference infant compares to a "male reference adult":

Component	Infant (3.5 kg, density 1.024 g/ml)	Adult (65.3 kg, density 1.064 g/ml)
	%	%
Water	75.1	62.4
Protein	11.4	16.1
Fat	11.0	15.3
Mineral	1.7	5.9
"Residue"	0.8	—
Fat-free body	89.0	84.7

During the twenty-year growing period there is a seventeen per cent decrease in total body water; protein and fat both increase by about forty per cent, and mineral by nearly two hundred fifty per cent. This, of course, represents the very significant increase in total skeletal mass: the mineralization of bones preformed in cartilage and the actual increase in size of most of the two hundred six bones that go to make up the adult skeleton.

There is a sex difference to be noted. In the newborn female fat forms a higher percentage, water a lower, of total body weight.

In a true sense, once we accept that body composition is made up of various tissue systems, which, in turn, are composed of varying combinations of minerals, proteins, etc., we can proceed to much more objective, more external, manifestations of growth. With height and weight established we may now consider the several contributions to over-all size made by major structural parts: the trunk, the arms, the legs.

The Trunk

The trunk, composed of head, neck, thoracic or lung cage, and abdomino-pelvic or visceral housing, is also known as the axial skeleton. It contributes largely to weight, for it has in infancy, seventy-five per cent of the body mass, and in later childhood, sixty-seven per cent. It also contributes about sixty to fifty per cent to stature, as stem length or sitting height. In infants the trunk is measured supine as crown-rump length (CR), from top of head to plane of buttocks when legs are flexed against abdomen. After two years of age it is measured as sitting height (SH) from top of head to plane of seat.

A newborn baby has a crown-rump/crown-sole index (CR/CS) of sixty to sixty-five per cent, i.e., that amount of total body length is in trunk. Between birth and five years the legs grow faster than the trunk and the index drops to about fifty-five per cent. At puberty the sex difference asserts itself, for trunk is relatively longer in girls (index of about fifty-two per cent), legs relatively longer in boys (index of about forty-eight per cent). This is why teen-age girls and adult females are "taller sitting down." In Figure 16, several trunk dimensions plus one

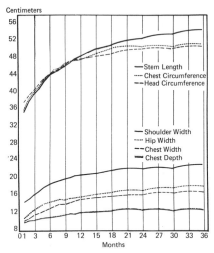

FIG. 16. Growth Curves, Birth to Three Years, of Seven Body Dimensions, Sexes Combined.

of the head, are shown from birth to three years, boys and girls combined. Noteworthy is the parallelism between growth of chest and head circumferences. Also note that stem length growth has a greater velocity than has other trunk dimensions, and that shoulder breadth is absolutely greater than hip width.

In Figure 17, stem length and breadth of shoulders, and in Figure 18, hip breadths are graphed from birth to twenty years (adult) for boys and girls. Stem length and shoulder breadth are absolutely larger in boys except for female dominance at 11:0–15:0. Hip breadth of boys exceeds that of girls in absolute size with the boys moving noticeably ahead at puberty. It is only *relatively* that a sex difference is to be seen, in the ratio hip B/shoulder B.

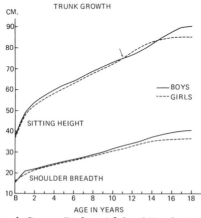

FIG. 17. Growth Curves, Birth to Adult, of Trunk Dimensions: Stem Length and Shoulder Breadth.

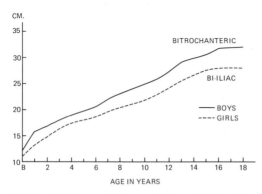

FIG. 18. Growth Curves, Birth to Adult, of Pelvic Breadths.

The girls have a higher index. If the trunk between shoulders and hips is regarded as a trapezoid the girls have the base at the hips, while in boys it is inverted, with base at shoulders. This is the "masculine build" of the adolescent boy, the "feminine build" of the adolescent girl.

The chest proportions change with age in that chest depth increases more rapidly than chest breadth, although the latter is absolutely the greater dimension. This change in proportion is seen in the *thoracic index* (chest breadth/ chest depth). At two years girls have a higher index than boys, but after that the boys catch up and they march along together until puberty when the index becomes higher in boys—more "deep-chested." All through growth Negro children have a chest "more flattened" in cross-section than do white children.

Arm and Leg

The arm and the leg together form what is called the "appendicular skeleton." Each limb is composed of three segments: arm = upper arm + lower arm or forearm + hand; leg = thigh + lower leg or shank + foot. Each segment has its own growth velocity, so that proportions change both intramembrally and intermembrally.

In the growth of the *arm* and its segments, the sexes parallel one another until puberty, at which time the boys forge ahead. The sex difference in total arm length is only ½″ until puberty; after that the boy's arm becomes 2½″ longer than the girls. The total arm length grows about 2.5 cm (1″) per year from age three to twelve years. The annual rate goes up to about 1½″ in boys, 1¼″ in girls during pubertal growth, then decelerates rapidly. Total arm length is greater in boys than girls, in Negroes than in whites. At birth the forearm is as long as the upper arm, but by adolescence the forearm L/upper arm L ratio is only about seventy-five per cent; it is higher in Negroes, i.e., they have a relatively longer forearm. During growth, hand length decelerates in rate relative to total arm length, i.e., the infant and young child have a relatively long hand. The Negro also has a longer arm relative to stature.

In the growth of the *leg* and its segments the sexes again parallel one another until puberty, at which time the boy's leg length becomes greater, both totally and segmentally. Changes in shank/thigh ratio parallel those of the forearm/upper arm ratio, i.e., thigh grows faster than shank. In Negro children the shank/thigh ratio is higher (relatively long shank). Also, the growth rates of arm and leg are such that total arm becomes relatively long compared to total leg.

It is interesting to observe that thigh and lower leg share in the "adolescent spurt" just as does stature. This is shown in Figure 19, where for fifty boys and fifty girls the velocity curves for stature, femur (thigh) and tibia (lower leg) are shown for ages eight to eighteen years. The timing of "peak" velocity is the same for stature,

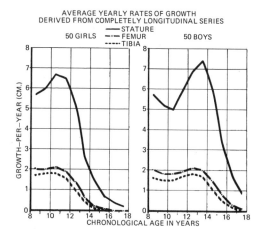

FIG. 19. Velocity Curves, 8–18 Years, for Lengths of Femur and Tibia.

femur, and tibia, within each sex, with girls two years ahead of boys.

The *circumferences* of the segments of the arm and leg may be noted for upper arm, forearm, and thigh (Figures 20 and 21). Forearm circumference in girls is less than in boys throughout growth, but thigh circumference is

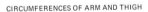

CIRCUMFERENCES OF ARM AND THIGH

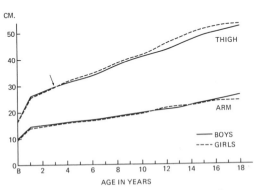

FIG. 20. Growth Curves, Birth to Adult, of Circumferences of Arm and Thigh.

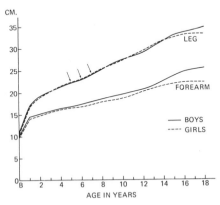

CIRCUMFERENCES OF FOREARM AND LEG

FIG. 21. Growth Curves, Birth to Adult, of Circumferences of Forearm and Leg.

greater from two years and on. Absolute and relative variability in size of circumference—a measure of the deposit of adipose tissue—increases in order of forearm to upper arm, to lower leg, to thigh. The velocity curve for circumference growth of all four segments, in both sexes, descends in the first year, increases to three years, and after five years has two "peaks," eleven to twelve years in girls, thirteen to fifteen years in boys.

In passing it may be noted that both arm and leg show the same secular increase in total length as does stature. Data on the arm show, for example, that the arm length of a 9:0 boy was on the average ½″ shorter in 1920 than in 1940. An 11:0 boy in 1955 had a leg longer by nearly 2″ (50 cm) than an 11:0 boy in 1890, and a thigh circumference 1¼″ (3.0 cm) greater.

The Foot

The *foot* merits extra consideration. After all, it is a distinctive human structure, for man is a biped—a "two-foot."

The prenatal growth of the foot goes something like this: at eight weeks length (L) = 0.2″, at three months L = 0.6″, at six months L = 2.0″, and at birth L = 3.2″ in boys, 3.1″ in girls.

Postnatally, in white boys, foot length grows from 3.2″ to 10.3″ (4:0″ at six months, 5.1″ at 18 months, 6.0″ at three years, 7.1″ at six years, 8.5″ at ten years, 10.0″ at sixteen years, 10:3″ as adult). From birth to ten years the white girl's foot is 0.1″ shorter than the boy's, but from 10–20 years it is 1″ shorter. However, the girls reach adult foot L values earlier: at birth the girl's foot L is thirty-four per cent of its adult value, the boy's thirty-one per cent; at ten years girls have ninety per cent of their adult foot L, the boys only eighty-two per cent. Foot L relative to stature is about 15.5% in boys, with a high of 15.9% at thirteen years, and about 14.5% in girls, with a high of 15.6% at ten years.

Children today are taller and have bigger feet, and girls get both stature and foot size earlier. That is why many mothers exclaim, "why, my daughter is only twelve years old, but already her shoe size is the same as mine!" True, but as an adult her feet will not be relatively large—she will grow up to them!

Negro children, on the average, have longer and broader feet. In both whites and Negroes the foot index (breadth/length) is fairly constant after the age of six years. Before that the foot was relatively broad.

The *arch* of the foot is a matter of concern to many parents. The problem has been tackled radiologically by Robinow and his colleagues, employing certain angular relationships in the foot bones. Figure 22 shows a high-arched foot, Figure 23, a low-arched foot. Most children's arches do not change much with age. Low arches are positively related to a high weight-for-height ratio, i.e., heavier children have a greater tendency to low arches.

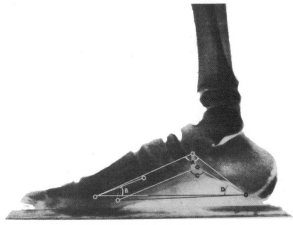

FIG. 22. X-ray Film of a High-Arched Foot.

If we accept the evidence of a high correlation in arch height between siblings, then there is probably a hereditary factor in high or low arch. Finally, a low arch is not

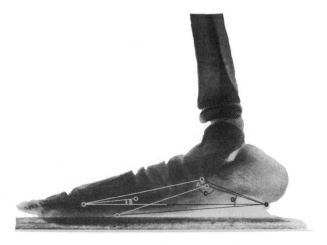

FIG. 23. X-ray Film of a Low-Arched Foot.

clearly related to knock-knees. Its role in posture will be discussed in Chapter X.

Body Fat

The circumference of an arm or leg segment, and of the trunk also, is made up—from the outside inward—of skin, subcutaneous fat, muscle, and bone. As a general rule, the greater the circumference the greater the amount of subcutaneous fat (though in postpubertal boys muscle may take precedence). There are two ways to measure fat: 1) by skinfolds; 2) radiographically, along with muscle and bone.

Before we go into methodology we should ask a few questions: "Why measure fat?"; "Why measure the fat-muscle-bone relationship?" The answer is that while height and weight are useful in following growth progress and in assessing the health and nutritional balance of not only a single child, but of different populations and different socio-economic groups, they are not enough. A heavy child may be a fat child, but he also may be heavy-muscled or large-boned. Contrariwise, an underweight child can be of a lean, linear build, or he may be poorly muscled or have slender, demineralized bones.

The simplest and the easiest estimation of fat is via *skinfolds*. With thumb and index finger a fold of skin + subcutaneous fat is pinched up and measured to the nearest 0.1 mm by a special "skinfold caliper." There are many sites where the measurement has been taken— under the chin, above the knee cap, below the shoulder blade, on the front of the chest just above the nipple (pre-pubescent), on the side of the chest wall, the back of the upper arm, the belly wall lateral to the navel, and the lateral crest of the pelvic girdle—but only two are neces-sary, for they tell the story adequately: 1) subscapular, just below the lowest point of the left shoulder blade; 2) tricipital, on the back of the left upper arm half-way between shoulder and elbow. These are the measurements that are used in the evaluation of the obese child.

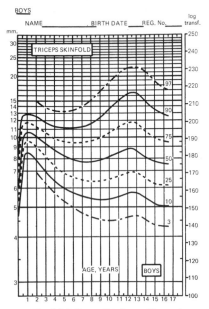

FIG. 24. Triceps Skinfold, Boys, Birth–17 Years (see text for details).

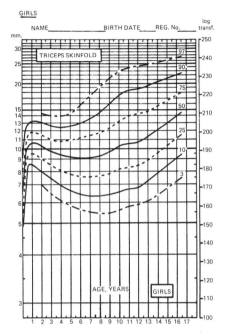

FIG. 25. Triceps Skinfold, Girls, Birth–17 Years (see text for details).

In Figures 24–27, are given the percentile values, from three per cent to ninety-seven per cent, for triceps and subscapular folds from birth to seventeen years in boys and girls. In both sexes there is a very rapid increase in both folds in the first year. In boys there is a decrease until about eight years, at which time a rapid increase begins (prepubertal spurt). In girls the triceps fold decreases a bit after infancy, then at five years begins a steady, even increase until seventeen years. The subscapular fold in both sexes increases steadily, with a slight dip in mid-childhood. Girls have a thicker subcutaneous fat layer at all ages past infancy, especially postpubertally. In the arm, for example, girls have twice as much fat as boys; but in boys the upper arm muscle mass doubles at adolescence.

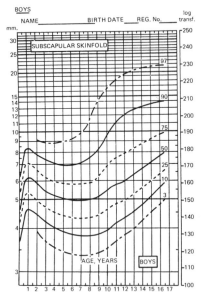

FIG. 26. Subscapular Skinfold, Boys, Birth–17 Years (see text for details).

In a study of 1,092 Philadelphia white and Negro children, age six to twelve years, the following race differences emerged: in general, Negroes have less subcutaneous fat; white girls have the highest skinfold measurements at all ages; white boys have thicker folds than Negro girls; the Negro girl has thicker skinfolds than the Negro boy.

Arm and Leg Compartments Via X-ray Film

By the use of serial antero-posterior X-ray films of the upper arm (mid-level) and the lower leg (greatest calf breadth) it is possible to watch how the *compartments* of the arm and leg grow, both relatively and absolutely. On the X-ray films, at the levels indicated, transverse measurements are taken: total breadth; skin + fat breadth; muscle breadth; bone breadth. These measurements give an insight into how the child's body—as seen in arm and

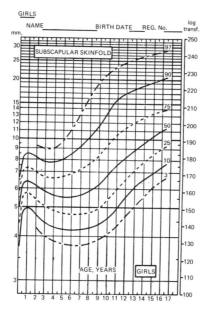

FIG. 27. Subscapular Skinfold, Girls, Birth–17 Years (see text for details).

leg—is composed, i.e., lean or fat, slender or stocky, muscular or not, big-boned or slender-boned, and so on. In a very objective way they give a real meaning to weight. As a rule the growth of the compartments follows a general growth curve. Before puberty fat increase is most highly correlated with weight; after puberty muscle is more highly correlated, most markedly in boys. At the age of one year total limb breadth, muscle, and bone are about sixty per cent of their adult value, while fat is about one hundred fifteen per cent, falling to sixty-five per cent at eight years. By fifteen years or so all compartments are ninety to ninety-five per cent of their adult value.

The measurement of fat, muscle, and bone relationships, when taken longitudinally in a child, has some prediction value. In girls, for example, who are fatter than average between eight and a half to nine and a half years, the onset of puberty will be earlier and the rate of skeletal maturity will be accelerated. In Figures 28–29, are shown, respectively, relative muscle and fat breadths (upper arm) in Philadelphia children, age six to fourteen years, who are *early, average,* and *late maturers.* In boys

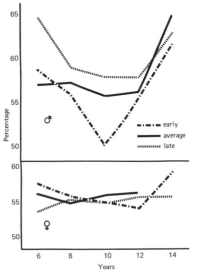

FIG. 28. Relative Muscle Breadth in Relation to Maturation.

it is the late maturers who are relatively well-muscled. The early-maturing boy, who will, on the average, be taller and heavier, does *not* have the muscle strength commensurate with his size. Just because he is bigger does not mean he is that much stronger. In girls relative muscle breadth shows no real difference by maturity class. For fat breadth the early maturing boys show a relatively much greater fat breadth at ten years. Again, maturity grouping in girls shows no significant difference. These findings are especially important for the early-maturing, fast-growing boy; he may be large for his age, but it is a fat-largeness rather than a muscle-largeness. There is every chance that his muscle-strength is a real laggard, compared to over-all body size.

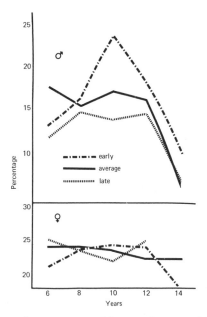

FIG. 29. Relative Fat Breadth in Relation to Maturation.

Muscle mass in infancy and early childhood is positively correlated with the development of motor behavior. Infants who stand alone, or who walk, at one year, are larger in leg muscle mass. There is probably a hereditary basis for tissue compartments as seen in Figure 30 for identical twins: there is virtual identity in calf muscle, bone, and fat in these girl twins, each followed between seven and a half to eleven and a half years of age.

Lean or Stocky Body-Build?

There is one final question in the consideration of tissue compartments: how do they throw light on over-all body-build from a linear (slender) to a lateral (stocky or fat) child?

In Figure 31 are depicted five "shape-types" developed by Tanner (1964) on the basis of five factors of build

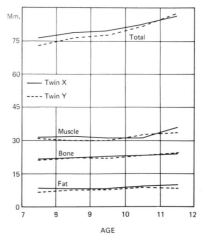

FIG. 30. Tissue Patterns (Bone, Muscle, Fat) in Identical Twins, 7–12 Years of Age (see text for details).

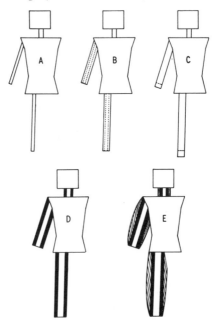

FIG. 31. Five "Shape Types," Based on Skeletal and Tissue Factors.

(A, B, and C are skeletal factors; D and E are soft tissue factors). In A the basis is average skeletal-size factors. In B all limb-bone breadths are above average (stockier). In C all limb-bone lengths are above average. In D muscle breadth has been added to bone breadths and lengths (big-boned, big-muscled). In E fat breadth has been added (this is the large "bulky" individual).

Thus in trunk and limbs we have seen that the growing child is a complex integration of physiological (functional) and morphological (structural) characteristics. They change with age, they change with rate of progress toward maturity, but always the changes are interrelated, for form and function unfold synchronously.

Jaws and Teeth

The theme of integrated growth is clearly seen in jaws and teeth for here two biological "ages" must work together: bone or skeletal age and tooth or dental age (both calcification and eruption times). In man, as in all mammals, the tooth, as it calcifies, forms its own socket; the original tooth nucleus is embedded in the jawbones—the maxillary bone above, the mandibular bone below. As each tooth gets larger, in its bony crypt, it erodes or resorbs the bone around it to form a closely fitting bony tooth-socket. This bone-tooth relationship means that bony jaws must get larger as the teeth get larger (the teeth calcify in order of cusps, crown, neck, and root). If, for some reason, there is a deviation in bone-growth timing and tooth-development timing, then a space problem may arise, i.e., crowding and possible malposition of teeth.

We have also in common with all mammals two sets of teeth: the "milk" or "baby" or deciduous set; and the permanent set. The first set is temporary, i.e., the first teeth fall out and are succeeded by the final set. There are twenty teeth in the first set, thirty-two in the second. In each set there are three or four different kinds of teeth;

two incisors, one canine, two milk molars in the first set; two incisors, one canine, two premolars, three molars in the second set. There are several ways of discussing or writing the first and second sets; in my work I prefer the following:

Tooth	*Deciduous*	*Permanent*
central incisor	i_1	I_1
lateral incisor	i_2	I_2
canine (cuspid)	c	C
first milk molar	m_1 ⎫	—
second milk molar	m_2 ⎬ *	—
first premolar (bicuspid)	—	P_1 ⎫
second premolar (bicuspid)	—	P_2 ⎬ *
first permanent molar	—	M_1 ⎫
second permanent molar	—	M_2 ⎬ **
third permanent molar	—	M_3 ⎭

*the milk molars are succeeded by the premolars.
**the permanent molars have no predecessors.

In order to differentiate lower and upper teeth we write like this: $\overline{M_1}$ or $\underline{M_1}$—the bar above the tooth shows it to be lower, while the bar below the tooth shows it to be upper. As a rule there is no reason except for purely dental purposes to differentiate right and/or left.

The eruption schedule of the first set of teeth is as follows:

	AVERAGE ERUPTION TIME			
Order	*7½ mos.*	*1 yr.*	*2 yrs.*	*3 yrs.*
Lower central incisor	+	+	+	+
Upper central incisor		+	+	+
Upper lateral incisor		+	+	+
Lower lateral incisor			+	+
Upper and lower first milk molar			+	+
Canine			+	+
Lower second milk molar				+
Upper second milk molar				+

There is, of course, individual variation—either earlier or later—in the above schedule. For example one study gives completion of the first teeth as 32–33 months for boys, 33–34 months for girls.

For the eruption schedule of the permanent teeth I am going to give two schedules: the first is from the Forsyth Dental Infirmary for Children, in Boston; the second is from the Fels Research Institute of Ohio (p. 82). The Forsyth schedule gives the mean and the range (±1 S.D. or sixteen per cent to eighty-four per cent).* The Fels schedule gives the range from the earliest five per cent to the latest five per cent (range of five per cent to ninety-five per cent).

If the baby teeth fall out too early—either by natural exfoliation or by accident—the pedodontist (children's dentist) should supervise this situation, trying to hold the space that is left to provide room for the permanent tooth to come in. If the baby teeth are held in place too long, again the pedodontist must take over, to find out the reason for the delay and then to proceed accordingly.

The first permanent tooth to erupt is the first molar, often referred to as the "six-year molar." Actually, this is no more than a rule of thumb that is almost folklore. This tooth may erupt any time between the ages of four and a half and eight, and still be entirely normal.

The third permanent molar is the so-called "wisdom tooth." Its presence or absence and its eruption are far too variable to give either average or range. "About twenty years" is as good a statement as any.

The foregoing outline of tooth eruption is not enough. The real problem comes when the teeth are erupted and when they are in place so that they can serve their function of biting and chewing. Then dental troubles, apart from decay, may begin! The teeth may "come in crooked" or be crowded or spaced, or they may be malaligned by various kinds of oral habits. It is estimated that about fifty per cent of American children have some kind or

*In the tabulation that follows I have called M − 1.S.D. *early* and M + 1.S.D. *late* in the Forsyth data.

PERMANENT TOOTH ERUPTION (YRS.)
(FORSYTH)

	BOYS			GIRLS		
Maxillary Teeth	*Early*	*Average*	*Late*	*Early*	*Average*	*Late*
Central incisor	6.67	7.47	8.25	6.38	7.20	8.00
Lateral incisor	7.67	8.67	9.67	7.21	8.20	9.17
Canine	10.33	11.69	13.08	9.63	10.98	12.33
First premolar	8.92	10.40	11.88	8.58	10.03	11.50
Second premolar	9.63	11.18	12.75	9.33	10.88	12.46
First molar	5.58	6.40	7.21	5.42	6.22	7.00
Second molar	11.33	12.68	14.04	10.92	12.27	13.63
Mandibular Teeth						
Central incisor	5.75	6.54	7.33	5.50	6.26	7.04
Lateral incisor	6.83	7.70	8.58	6.46	7.34	8.21
Canine	9.50	10.79	12.08	8.58	9.86	11.13
First premolar	9.33	10.82	12.29	8.71	10.18	11.67
Second premolar	9.79	11.47	13.17	9.21	10.89	12.58
First molar	5.42	6.21	7.00	5.13	5.94	6.75
Second molar	10.75	12.12	13.50	10.29	11.66	13.00

PERMANENT TOOTH ERUPTION (YRS.)
(FELS)

	BOYS		GIRLS	
Maxillary Teeth	*Early* (5%)	*Late* (95%)	*Early* (5%)	*Late* (95%)
Central incisor	5.9	9.1	5.6	8.8
Lateral incisor	6.8	10.6	6.3	10.1
Canine	9.0	14.4	8.3	13.7
First premolar	7.5	13.3	7.2	12.9
Second premolar	8.1	14.3	7.8	14.0
First molar	4.8	8.0	4.7	7.8
Second molar	10.0	15.4	9.6	15.0
Mandibular Teeth				
Central incisor	5.0	8.1	4.7	7.8
Lateral incisor	6.0	9.6	5.6	9.1
Canine	8.3	13.3	7.4	12.4
First premolar	7.9	13.7	7.8	13.1
Second premolar	8.2	14.8	7.6	14.2
First molar	4.4	7.8	4.4	7.5
Second molar	9.5	14.8	9.0	14.3

degree of malocclusion (bad relationship between teeth of upper and lower dental arches, or within each arch).

Oral Habits and Malocclusion

The problem of oral habits—thumb or finger sucking, the use of a pacifier, mouth breathing, lip sucking and/or biting, and so on—is a difficult and variable one. Usually three sets of reasons are given for thumb and/or finger sucking: 1) reflex, either fetal or in infancy, due to the fact that touching or stroking the lips evokes a sensory-motor response, most frequently met by inserting thumb or finger; 2) frustration of an oral drive, either innate or learned (here enters the question of breast-feeding, pro or con, duration, etc.); 3) psychological stress, either parent-child or child-sibling. Each one of these sets of factors, or any combination, may be causative in a given child; variations in kind and degree are almost infinite.

How frequent is "digital" sucking (thumb and/or finger)? This is difficult to answer. An Australian study noted a forty-five per cent frequency in a pediatric practice, nineteen per cent in respiratory clinic patients, and fourteen per cent in an orthodontic practice. These are not random samples, so that the range of forty-five per cent to fourteen per cent tells little.

What can or should be done about digital sucking? This, too, is hard to answer. The same Australian study, carried over an eight-year period, found in twenty-one children who persisted in the habit for at least eight years, that family nagging, talks with a physician or dentist, and the use of preventives (either chemical or mechanical) were all of no avail.

There are quite a few American psychologists and orthodontists who feel that thumb or index finger sucking is not harmful. It is a sort of "tranquilizing habit" often resorted to only at bedtime. Most children stop of their own accord at about two or three years of age.

The problem of malocclusion must be briefly considered. The kinds of malocclusion are defined in three main types, called "Classes": Class I, with upper and lower first permanent molar in good front-to-back alignment, but anterior teeth crowded or otherwise malpositioned; Class II, with lower first permanent molar backward in position relative to upper first permanent molar to give a retruded or receding lower face (lower jaw); Class III, with lower first permanent molar forward in position relative to upper first permanent molar to give a protruded lower face (lower jaw). There are subtypes of these classes but that is a matter for the orthodontist to determine.

The American Association of Orthodontists has listed a number of *causes of malocclusion.* I shall mention them as follows:

1. Heredity: this usually involves the idea that the child inherits, for example, the "large teeth" of the father, the "small jaws" of the mother. I have not found this to be demonstrated in over three thousand case-histories of malocclusion. Class III ("undershot" lower jaw) does seem to run in families, as, for example, the "Hapsburg jaw." About all I am prepared to say is that the likelihood of a malocclusion in a given case is heightened if there is a family background (in either the father's or the mother's line) of malocclusion, lessened if there is not.

2. Missing teeth: this refers to congenitally missing teeth, i.e., teeth that never did form. In such cases there are bound to be problems of tooth-spacing and arch relationships.

3. Supernumerary or extra teeth: these are due, usually, to some kind of reduplication of the thirty-two permanent teeth or the twenty deciduous teeth. They create spacing (crowding) problems; also, if they are present in either dentition, they may delay eruption of the normal twenty or thirty-two teeth.

4. Abnormal frenum: this is in the mid-line and is a gumlike strip of tissue usually between the upper cen-

tral incisors; it may cause spacing problems. (Some geneticists feel that the spacing between the upper central incisors is hereditary.)

5. Pressure from sleeping or posture habits: sleeping with hand under the face may cause a right- or left-sided jaw asymmetry; there is appearing a "TV Syndrome," involving the child who lies on his belly to watch TV, supporting his head by cupping his lower jaw in his hands—this pushes the lower jaw back and may result in a Class II-like receding jaw.

6. Thumb-sucking: this habit, if indulged to excess, may push the upper front teeth out ("bucking" them), the lower teeth in, to give an excessive overjet, i.e., the upper anterior teeth project markedly in front of the lower anterior teeth. Many orthodontists feel that thumb-sucking is a factor only when there is already a slight malocclusion. In other words, it "makes a bad matter worse."

7. Tongue thrust: due to a peculiar swallowing pattern wherein the tongue pushes forward between the front teeth as the child swallows. This forces the upper and lower jaws apart to give an "anterior open bite." The tongue habit must be alleviated, under orthodontic supervision, before the bite can be closed.

8. Premature shedding or loss of the deciduous teeth: unless the vacated space is retained, the permanent successors may be malaligned; similarly, if permanent teeth are lost too soon—especially the first permanent molars—the space must be retained lest the second premolars drift backward or the second permanent molars drift forward.

9. Prolonged retention of deciduous teeth: this may cause a malrelationship in the eruption of the permanent teeth, either with reference to sequence or to spacing.

10. Mouth breathing: this may lead to a high, narrow-arched palate, with resultant crowding; however, not all mouth breathers have a malocclusion.

I shall not discuss *facial growth* in detail, beyond saying that the head and face, like the rest of the body,
grows in three dimensions: height, breadth, depth. In the
face *height* is vertical from root of nose to chin; *breadth*
is transverse, across the cheek-bones and across the jaw
angles; *depth* is sagittal or anterior-posterior, in that the
face literally grows forward in relation to the skull (the
brain-box).

There is order in facial growth, just as there is order in
bodily growth. For the face I have derived the formula
4–5½–7, for growth in breadth, height, and depth dimensions, respectively. Here is how it works out: when the
child is born his facial breadth dimensions are sixty per
cent of his adult size, his facial heights forty-five per cent,
and his facial depths thirty per cent. This means that forty
per cent of facial breadths growth is postnatal, fifty-five
per cent of facial heights, seventy per cent of his facial
depths. Hence, postnatally the face grows least in breadth
(the *4*), next in height (the *5½*), and most in depth (the
7). As this 4–5½–7 pattern unfolds normally the bone-
tooth relationship is more apt to be good and the likelihood of malocclusion correspondingly reduced. If, for any
reason, the 4–5½–7 pattern is out of balance—either in
amount or timing—then the likelihood of malocclusion is
correspondingly increased. In a certain number of cases a
disharmonious growth interplay between height, breadth
and depth dimensions may set up a malocclusion due to
a tooth-bone discrepancy (usually severe crowding).

With this chapter concludes the discussion of what may
be termed almost purely *structural growth:* height,
weight, the areas of the total body, the makeup of the
body and its parts, and a final look at the head-face-tooth
complex. In other words we are through with *form.* Now
we must look at *function.* First, what the growing human
body is; next, what "makes it tick."

ENDOCRINE GLANDS AND GROWTH

The Hormones of the Body

In the first five chapters of this book I have dealt with what may be considered as the external manifestations of growth, i.e., changes in size, in proportion, in compartmentalization, in skeletal maturation, and so on. All of this is objective and is easily quantifiable. The integrated result is, of course, growth of bone, muscle, organs, and various tissues to make up total bodily growth.

The processes of growth are not random, but are, to speak in computer terms, programmed. This "programming," as we shall see, goes back ultimately to the genetic code; in a sense genetics is a "pre-determiner" for it establishes each child's pattern of growth. However, the unfolding of that pattern is monitored by a host of environmental factors. Growth progress is governed by a complex system of checks and balances, both inner—within the total organism itself—and outer—the sum of the situations within which the individual grows and matures.

As a heritage from age-old vertebrate and mammalian ancestors we have in our bodies a number of glands of internal secretion or endocrine glands, secretions of which are known as *hormones*. Broadly, a hormone is a chemical substance, released into the blood stream by a cell or group of cells, which produces a physical effect on other body cells. The secretion of a given endocrine gland is specific for certain end-cells.

Hormones have a number of functions: 1) they regulate the tempo or pace of bodily function, or metabolism (as examples, the thyroid for the basal or over-all bodily metabolic rate, the parathyroid for utilization of calcium, the pancreas for utilization of carbohydrates, the adrenal for balance in the body of sodium, potassium, and water); 2) they preside over structural increase or growth; 3) they establish basic sex differences, set the sex drive, and regulate reproduction; 4) they influence the nervous system, facilitate mental processes, and hence make for personality differences; 5) they may aid in the manufacture of antibodies for immunization against the pathology of disease. In short, hormones are fundamental to many life processes, and are basic to life itself.

In Figure 32 are shown outline drawings of a male and female body. Drawn in, and correctly located, are the many endocrine glands.

It is not an overstatement to say that each gland and its hormone(s) has something to do with growth, some more than others. In this chapter I shall limit discussion to what I deem the four major endocrine glands involved in bodily growth: the pituitary, the thyroid, the adrenal, and the gonad or sex glands (testis, ovary).

To discuss each of these four singly is a tour de force, for each is related to the other not only directly but also indirectly via a feedback mechanism. Endocrine action and reaction are interrelated, not single. Nowhere is this better exemplified than for the pituitary, often called the "master gland of the body."

The Pituitary and the Growth Hormone

In Figure 33, Dr. Choh Hao Li, of the University of California, has portrayed the ways in which the pituitary affects other glands, especially thyroid, adrenal, testis, and ovary. (The pituitary has three lobes: anterior, mid

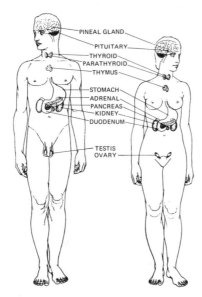

PINEAL GLAND
PITUITARY
THYROID
PARATHYROID
THYMUS
STOMACH
ADRENAL
PANCREAS
KIDNEY
DUODENUM
TESTIS
OVARY

FIG. 32. The Endocrine Glands of Male and Female.

or intermediate, and posterior. Dr. Li shows only the hormones of the anterior lobe.) There is one that stands out for us, viz., the growth hormone, for somatic or bodily growth.

Just what does the anterior lobe of the pituitary do? For what structures and/or functions is it responsible? I venture to list its growth-oriented chores as follows: 1) it produces the growth hormone (HGH) which, as the term implies, is responsible for size increases; 2) it promotes, in the female, breast development and milk production; 3) it regulates ovarian and testicular function (ovulation and female sex hormone or estrogen, and sperm and male sex hormone, or androgen); 4) it stimulates the thyroid to secrete thyroxin; 5) it stimulates the cortex or outer layer of the adrenal to secrete an androgenic hormone (in both sexes). The hormones, orchestrated in a symphony of growth and maturation, are the prime mov-

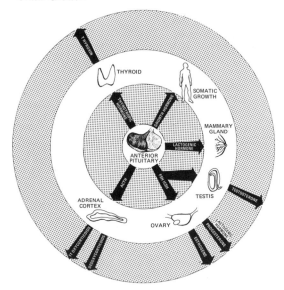

FIG. 33. Anterior Portion of the Pituitary Gland in Relation to Other Endocrine Glands.

ers in all the bodily changes that occur in the twenty-year growing period. Of these changes those of the skeleton give us the most useful and objective ratings of growth in "amount" and rate.

If you, the reader, will roll back the tip of your tongue to the roof of your mouth (as far back as you can), then you will have located a significant area. Straight up from the rolled-up tongue-tip, at the base of the brain, is the pituitary gland; right above it is not only the brain itself, but a very specific part or area of the brain, the *hypothalamus.* In this hypothalamus is a structure called the *median eminence.* Here are to be found "releasing factors," which are compounds of low molecular weight. These compounds are secreted from neurones (nerve cells) in the region of the median eminence, and enter into the anterior pituitary portal blood system.

Via the releasing factor it is the brain that controls certain endocrine systems, viz., the growth hormone, the gonadal stimulating hormones, the thyroid stimulating hormone, and the adrenal stimulating hormone (adrenocorticotrophic hormone, or ACTH). All these hormones have been extracted in pure form, and one—that to the thyroid—has been synthesized.

Growth Promotion

Out of the complex and numerous kinds of hormones comes an oft-asked question: in children who are extremely "short for age," is it possible to make the (boy) (girl) grow taller? (Usually a boy is involved.) There is one thing to be said at once: the shortness or "dwarfing" *must* be due to an endocrine insufficiency, often hypopituitary or hypothyroid, i.e., insufficient growth hormone or thyroxin. A very frequent cause of short stature is childhood diabetes, due to insufficiency of insulin secretion. However, here there is often a genetic factor, and hence the condition is both hereditary (genetic) and environmental (faulty pancreatic function). Children with diabetes often are short as adults, though within normal range of variation.

The therapeutic administration of either the growth hormone or thyroxin will stimulate growth but *not beyond the child's inherited size potential.* In 1957 researchers at the University of California reported on the growth stimulation of seventy-two short, immature boys; fifty-nine were treated with a male sex hormone (methyltestosterone) and thirteen with the same hormone + thyroxin. As a group, their skeletal age was 17.4 months *behind* their chronological age. Before treatment their adult height prediction averaged 66″ (5′6″), with S.D. = 3.9″. The average dosage of the hormone used was 10 mg per day.

The results were moderately favorable[*] for height, and

[*]A useful index and a method of calculating relative rate in treated cases is to take stature at beginning and end of the period of treatment and express the height as follows:

very favorable in terms of maturation. The boys averaged 1.1″ *taller* than predicted, i.e., a little over 5′7″ instead of 5′6″. On the other hand a pubertal acceleration was achieved without accelerating skeletal age beyond chronological age. The prime results were psychological, in that sexual maturation was achieved. In cases such as these the best time for treatment is at an age when the circumpubertal acceleration would normally occur.

I have worked with very short children and the three most frequent groups that present themselves are mainly as follows: 1) children, most often boys, who are "short normals"; they are at or below the fifth percentile for stature for age and sex and there is a history of familial shortness; 2) children who are of the same percentile ranking, but who had a birth weight of 4½ lbs, or less (they are not necessarily prematures); 3) finally, of course, children who are far behind in stature because of insufficiency of the growth hormone, and/or inadequate response of peripheral tissue to endocrine stimulation.

At the University of London, Tanner and his associates studied children grouped much as above. All showed retardation in S.A. or bone age: 1.9 years in the "short normals," 1.3 years in the birth under-weight, and 2.7 years in the growth hormone failures; the ratio of S.A. to C.A. was seventy-one per cent, seventy-five per cent, fifty-seven per cent, respectively. Skinfold thicknesses were much greater in the third or endocrine group, even though this group was more than 3 S.D. *below* the average in stature.

In a sample of twenty-six short-statured children, sixteen of whom were hypopituitary dwarfs, ranging in age from 2.1–19.4 years, HGH was administered. All were

---

$\dfrac{\text{Ht. at end} - \text{Ht. at beginning}}{\text{av. Ht.}}$ + period of treatment as a decimal of year.

Example: boy grows from 103 cm to 109 cm in six months:

$$\frac{109 - 103}{106} \times \frac{1}{0.50} = \frac{6}{53} = 11.3\% \text{ per year.}$$

measured every three months before treatment began, and all were under treatment for at least one year. The HGH dosage varied, mainly because of unequal strength of the several batches received. In a subgroup of ten who were hyposomatropic (not enough growth hormones) and who responded well, the average pre-treatment height velocity was 0.52 times that expected; in the first year of treatment it was 1.92 times that expected; in the second year seven of the ten had a height growth velocity 1.62 times that expected. The S.A. also "caught up," but not as much as did stature. Two of the twenty-six were normal small children (familial), and did *not* respond to HGH.

The failure to respond to HGH poses a real problem. Essentially, the introduction of the HGH is similar to that of the introduction of any "foreign body." The tissues may react to this situation by the manufacture of an "antibody" which, in effect, combats or counteracts the effect of the substance introduced. This occasionally happens in a child given HGH—it just doesn't "take," with the result that expected growth stimulation is not achieved.

The change in skinfold thickness that occurred merits comment. Where the height response was good in HGH therapy, in children low in the growth hormone, the triceps and subscapular skinfold values decreased and muscle mass (volume) increased. In normal children there is fat increase until nine months, then decrease. The question: is this decrease due to a take-over of the growth hormone? Retarded height growth often shows up in the first year of life, and in these cases the skinfold thickness does not increase. Again, at the time of the adolescent height spurt, fat does not increase. There is a tie-up between fat decrease (or fat mobilization) and HGH sufficiency and fat persistence and HGH inadequacy. This relationship is not necessarily cause-and-effect, but may well represent two possible alternating effects of a more generalized growth process.

Dwarfism

The end results of the growth hormone have over the years attracted the public imagination. Too little of its outpouring produces dwarfs, too much produces giants. There have been several pituitary dwarfs of historic note. John Jarvis was a 21″ tall page to Queen Mary of England. Jeffery Hudson (1619–1682) was an 18″ tall page to the Duke of Buckingham, who once entertained Charles I by having Jeffery pop out of a pie set before the King. Richebourg, 23″ tall, was a French dwarf who died in 1858, at the age of ninety.

The best-known of the pituitary dwarfs was "General Tom Thumb" (Charles Stratton) of the mid-1800's in the United States. Tom was 3′2″ tall and was managed by the famous P. T. Barnum (see Figure 34). One of

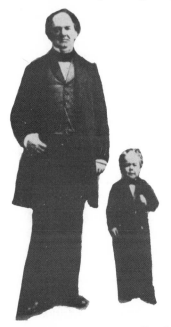

FIG. 34. P. T. Barnum and Tom Thumb.

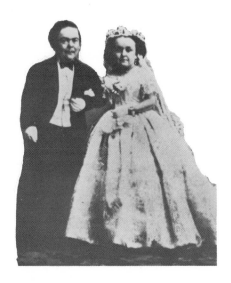

FIG. 35. Tom Thumb and His Wife Lavinia.

the most famous marriages of the nineteenth century was Tom's to the 2'8" Lavinia Bump (also known as Lavinia Warren) on February 10, 1863; (see Figure 35). It is not clear if they had children (even though for publicity purposes, the astute Barnum provided a borrowed few as evidence), but it is known that Lavinia's sister, also a midget, died in childbirth.

There are many types of dwarfism other than endocrine, the causes of which are many and varied: 1) *skeletal abnormalities,* of which achondroplasia is the most common and which is genetic, due to a single dominant autosomal gene; these dwarfs have normal heads and trunks but disproportionately very short arms and legs; rickets may cause rachitic dwarfism; 2) *nutritional* dwarfism, due to mal- or under-nutrition, either pre- or postnatal; failure to absorb ingested food is included here, as in coeliac disease (failure to handle proteins); 3) dwarfism due to *abnormalities of the central nervous system,* with encephalitis as a well-known, though not too common, cause; 4) *metabolic* dwarfism, including inborn errors of metabolism; here, for example, is included Vitamin D-resistant rickets; 5) *other systemic failures,* involving lungs, kidney, liver, and circulatory disorders; 6) *chronic anemia;* 7) *chronic infection and parasitism;* 8) *inadequate familial care,* especially mother-child;* 9) *other causes,* usually involving genetic failure (often multi-genetic failure), i.e., the dwarfism is but one phase or aspect of a variety of systemic (structural and/or functional) anomalies.

The Thyroid

Nearly every organ system in the body may be altered by an insufficiency of the thyroid hormone, thyroxin, for it has a major effect on oxygen consumption, that is, it stimulates the oxygen intake of virtually every tissue in the body. It promotes protein metabolism and increases the formation of the chemical which regulates muscle energy. It is also involved in the regulation of fat, carbohydrate, water, and mineral metabolism.

Thyroid dwarfism (hypothyroid) and pituitary dwarfism (hypopituitary) are often combined, to a degree; indeed there are endocrinologists who speak of "hypopituitarythyroidism" and "hypothyropituitarism," the first-named in each category being a primary factor, the last-named, a secondary factor.

As mentioned before, an achondroplastic dwarf has a disproportionate body, with "normal" head and trunk, very short arms and legs. In contrast to the achondroplast the pituitary dwarf is well proportioned. This does not hold true for the thyroid dwarf especially if the child is thyroid deficient at birth (a cretin). In these children there is a generalized failure in both size and proportion.

---

*Here the child may become so emotionally involved that there results a *functional* hypopituitarism.

Infantile proportions persist with long trunk and short limbs, especially noticeable in the leg; in some severe cases the outward appearance is similar to that of an achondroplast.

Maturation processes are greatly retarded: bone development is such that the growing ends of the long bones which should unite with the shaft by about twenty years or so, remain un-united for a varying period of time, stated by some to reach into the forty to fifty year decade.

The administration of thyroxin stimulates both growth and maturation. In Figure 36 is seen a hypothyroid female

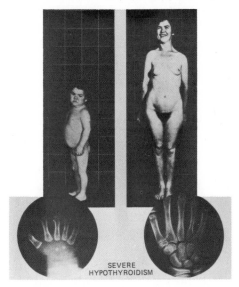

FIG. 36. Hypothyroidism: Left, 10 Years of Age; Right, 18 Years of Age.

dwarf at age ten before treatment, and at age eighteen, after treatment. At ten years (left) her height was only 35.5″ (normal 54″) and her hand-wrist bone age was only six months (9:6 retarded). At eighteen her height was 60″ (normal 64″) and her bone age was 14:0 (a gain of 13:6 in eight years, now only 4:0 retarded). She not only grew, but she became sexually mature. The thyroxin evidently not only greatly improved the metabolic balance, but it had a pronounced feedback effect on anterior pituitary: the secretion of the growth hormone was heightened so that she grew 24.5″; likewise, the secretion of sex-stimulating hormones was heightened to produce the evident development of secondary sex traits.

The hyperthyroid child is in marked contrast to the hypothyroid child:

Trait	Hypothyroid	Hyperthyroid
Size	Dwarfed	Normal
Proportions	Infantile	Normal
General appearance and behavior	Dull, lethargic	Normal (may be hyperkinetic, to a degree)
Mentality	Retarded	Normal
Basal metabolic rate (BMR)	Low	High
Bone development	Retarded	Normal

A thyroid dwarf given thyroxin must be carefully followed, checked at least at three-month intervals, especially when the chronological age is within normal circumpubertal range (say, the ten to sixteen year period). The thyroid hormone stimulates growth, as has been noted, but it may accelerate skeletal maturation faster than skeletal growth. In other words it hastens maturation of growing end and shaft which means, in conjunction with the sex hormone, cessation of linear bone growth. Hence, it is possible that thyroid administration may defeat itself, in the sense that unduly hastened long-bone union may be a height-retardant.

The Adrenal

The adrenal gland has basically an outer cortex and an inner medulla: the former develops from mesoderm cells in the sixth embryonic week; the latter from nerve tissue ectodermal cells in the seventh week. The cortex produces *steroid* hormones, the medulla produces hormones which influence blood pressure and pulse rate and which act upon peripheral blood vessels. There are three groups of steroid hormones: 1) those which maintain water, sodium, and potassium balance; 2) those which maintain the carbohydrate-protein balance; 3) and those which promote masculinization and nitrogen retention; and are found in the urine as a chemical called 17-ketosteroid, which from birth to eight years is in negligible amounts, but which thereafter regularly increase in amount to puberty.

With no intention of being irreverent I would modify "male and female created He them," to "androgen and estrogen created He them." These two hormones are the very essence of maleness and femaleness, respectively, in all of the animal kingdom. Figure 37 shows the male and

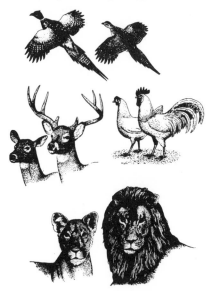

FIG. 37. Maleness and Femaleness in Birds and Mammals.

female pheasant, deer, chicken, and lion. The plumage of the female pheasant is due to the estrogen, while androgens are the cause of the rooster's comb and spur, the buck deer's antlers, and the lion's mane; remembering, of course, that the endocrines in these animals act in concert with the specific genetic make-up of each.

The Gonads

The gonads—testis in the male, ovary in the female—play a very important role in growth and maturation. The hormonal secretion of the gonads is influenced by the sex-stimulating hormone of the anterior pituitary. They are found in the urine along with the earliest sign of puberty (increase in gonad size), but recently it has been stated that traces were found in the urine as early as two years. In Figure 38 are shown age changes in the excretion of sex hormones.* In the male the androgens are both testicular and adrenal, in the female they are basically adrenal. The estrogens in the female are ovarian, while in the male they arise from vestigial structures in the urinogenital system. In both sexes the rise in endocrine excretion oc-

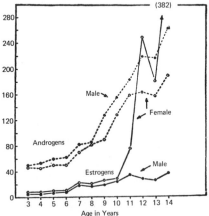

FIG. 38. The Secretion of Androgens and Estrogens in Males and Females in Relation to Age.

*The androgens (17-ketosteroids) are expressed in arbitrary color units, the estrogens in international units. See N. W. Shock, "Physiological Changes in Adolescence," in *Adolescence,* ed. W. B. Henry (1944), p. 75.

curs in the transition period between mid- and late childhood, i.e., around the tenth year.

The male androgenic hormone, testosterone, is a biologically more potent androgen than is the adrenal androgen. The testicular androgens have metabolic effects: they promote protein synthesis, muscle development, bone growth and final union of growing end and shaft, and govern the growth of primary and secondary sex apparatuses. Testosterone is derived from the Leydig cells of the testis, and is stimulated by a hormone of the anterior pituitary. Spermatogenesis occurs within the testicular tubules and is stimulated by another hormone of the anterior pituitary. Spermatogenesis is completed two to three years *after* the onset of puberty.

The *ovary* primarily secretes estrogen (estradiol-17) and progesterone, and secondarily a small amount of androgen. Estradiol-17 is biologically the most potent. The estrogens are stimulated by a hormone of the anterior pituitary. The principal metabolic effects of estrogen are as follows: 1) under certain circumstances it will influence protein metabolism; 2) it presides over linear growth and maturation; 3) it regulates time and nature of primary and secondary sex characteristics; 4) at puberty it affects fat metabolism, along with the adrenal corticoids, to give the female body its definitive configuration; 5) breast development, the earliest sign of puberty in the girl, is mediated by estrogen + progesterone, while lactation is affected by the growth hormone and prolactin, both from the anterior pituitary. The menstrual cycle is regulated by hormones from the anterior pituitary.

Gonadal maldevelopment occurs, typically, when the embryogenic gonad has not structurally differentiated as it should. Such cases are often linked with chromosomal aberrations.

In gonadal failure (castration) before puberty in the male, sexual maturity does not occur and the voice does not change. The individual is tall, slender, often very long-legged ("stork-legged"), with poor muscle development; often "breasts" develop. If castration occurs after puberty is attained, stature and proportions do not change; here, too, "breasts" often develop; the bones become osteoporotic or demineralized.

In gonadal failure due to developmental failure of the embryogenic tissue of the ovary the hypofunction delays puberty and sexual maturation. If the ovarian failure is postpubertal, menstruation ceases, the secondary female sex traits regress (breasts especially), the sex drive is greatly diminished, the bones become demineralized or osteoporotic, and "hot flashes" and emotional instability often ensue.

As may be seen in Figure 32 there are several hormones not considered in this chapter. They are all vital to the efficient functioning of the body, of course, but in the total growth process they are supplementary or complementary, rather than basic.

VII

PUBERTY AND ADOLESCENCE

What Is an Adolescent?

Growth in the second decade of life, encompassing both puberty and adolescence, is at once as dramatic and, in a way, as traumatic, as is birth. At birth we are launched into *all* life, with *all* of its potential. Sometime between ten and twenty years we come to fruition, for the potential becomes more real: we are brought to the threshold of full maturity with all of its rights and privileges, and all of its responsibilities. Puberty is a biological ripening. Adolescence is a behavioral-cultural ripening. With both we cross new frontiers, enter new worlds. Of the two, puberty, even though it be relatively a brief growth-moment, presents the greater changes. It may be said that puberty is organic, adolescence is experiential.

Adolescence is defined as "the period between puberty and maturity" by *Gould's Medical Dictionary. The Oxford Standard Dictionary* is more precise, defining it as "the period between childhood and maturity, extending from fourteen to twenty-five years in males, twelve to twenty-one years in females." Shock calls it a period of "physiological learning." Gallagher says it is "a state or process of growing up from childhood to manhood or womanhood." I prefer to regard it as "an adjustive, behavioral transition between puberty and adulthood." Adolescence is a time of ferment: the yeasting of body

103

chemistry and of socio-behavioral functioning. It is a time of triumph and a period of doubt, a time of realization and a period of uncertainty. It is an end and a beginning: an end of dependent acceptance and a beginning of self-determination. It is a seismic period in the life of the growing child—*and* of many of those around him! It lies between the eventide of childhood and the dawn of adulthood, with too often an in-between period of darkness.

I venture to suggest that adolescence may play a major role in the child's mental health: if there are wounds of an earlier childhood they may be healed by the richness of full self-realization, or they can be inflamed and deepened by the frustrations of a feeling of self-inadequacy.

Adolescence is truly "a brave new world" in almost every aspect of human growth biology, and in many aspects of personal-social adjustment to age- and sex-peer groups and to society at large.

In both sexes the onset of the outward pubertal changes is triggered by the beginning of accelerated height growth, the so-called "adolescent spurt." If serial data on the child are kept, it will be remembered that this is the marked upswing in the velocity curve for height (see Figure 7). The upswing occurs sometime in the ten-to-fifteen-year period, a year or two earlier in girls. Then, for the next three or four years the sequential metamorphosis into manhood and womanhood takes place.

Events of Puberty: Boy

As is true of all traits of physical growth, whether dimensional or descriptive, there is a sequence and there is a time. *Both are variable!* It is impossible to give an average age-order to the entire process of achieving sexual maturity. In general I venture to state three major growth-phases in the adolescent cycle: I. the onset of the height spurt; II. age of maximum height spurt; III. achievement of adult height.

In the boy the major sex-changes revolve around genital growth (testes, penis, scrotum), body hair development (axillary, pubic, facial, arms, legs, chest, head), voice change, and the more subtle changes in bearing (total facial appearance and general bodily carriage). The following "flow-chart" (p. 106) lists twenty male sex characteristics which are reasonably in order. The numbers in parentheses are in years and are mid-values for each trait. Within the sequence of twenty there may be time-shifts of ± one year.

Within a year or so of the beginning of accelerated height growth the male genitals begin to grow in size: the penis will grow longer and will increase in circumference; the testes will grow larger and as they do, the scrotum will get larger, will become wrinkled or furrowed, and will be increasingly pigmented; the temperature of the scrotum will average 2° less than that of the body generally; the prostate gland will increase in size and will secrete; at about twelve and a half years increased amounts of androgen (as 17-ketosteroid) will be found in the urine. At this time pubic, axillary, facial, and body hairs will begin the progressive unfolding of their respective patterns. Height growth will attain its maximum velocity in the early genital and hair changes. Finally, at an average of seventeen and three quarters years, stature, proportions, and total sex development will be achieved: boyhood meets manhood!

In a more or less summary form we may recognize five classificatory stages in male genital and pubic hair development. For each stage, I venture to give an average age and its normal range of variation. Thus, Stage II is (12 ± 1), which means that normally two of every three boys will attain this stage between 11–13 years.

Stage I. Penis, testes, scrotum, as in midchildhood; only fine down hair is to be found on the entire body.

I. *Onset of Height Spurt* (10–11)

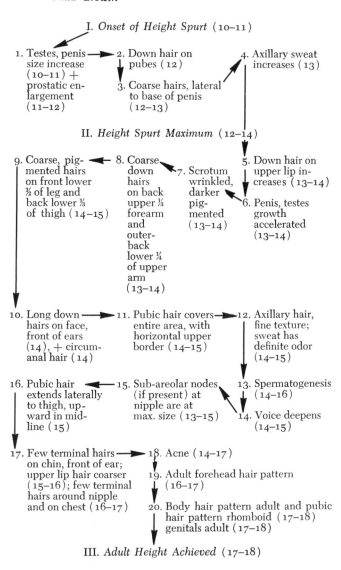

1. Testes, penis → 2. Down hair on   4. Axillary sweat
   size increase   pubes (12)   increases (13)
   (10–11) +
   prostatic en-   3. Coarse hairs, lateral
   largement   to base of penis
   (11–12)   (12–13)

II. *Height Spurt Maximum* (12–14)

9. Coarse, pig- ← 8. Coarse   5. Down hair on
   mented hairs   down ←7. Scrotum   upper lip in-
   on front lower   hairs   wrinkled,   creases (13–14)
   ½ of leg and   on back darker
   back lower ⅓   upper ⅓ pig-   6. Penis, testes
   of thigh (14–15) forearm mented   growth
                      and   (13–14)   accelerated
                      outer-   (13–14)
                      back
                      lower ¼
                      of upper
                      arm
                      (13–14)

10. Long down → 11. Pubic hair covers → 12. Axillary hair,
    hairs on face,   entire area, with   fine texture;
    front of ears   horizontal upper   sweat has
    (14), + circum- border (14–15)   definite odor
    anal hair (14)   (14–15)

16. Pubic hair ← 15. Sub-areolar nodes   13. Spermatogenesis
    extends laterally   (if present) at   (14–16)
    to thigh, up-   nipple are at
    ward in mid-   max. size (13–15) 14. Voice deepens
    line (15)   (14–15)

17. Few terminal hairs → 18. Acne (14–17)
    on chin, front of ear;
    upper lip hair coarser 19. Adult forehead hair pattern
    (15–16); few terminal   (16–17)
    hairs around nipple
    and on chest (16–17) 20. Body hair pattern adult and pubic
                                hair pattern rhomboid (17–18)
                                genitals adult (17–18)

III. *Adult Height Achieved* (17–18)

Grouping
Traits 1, 6, 14, 15, 20 are morphological (structural)
Traits 2, 3, 8, 9, 10, 11, 12, 16, 17, 20 are body hair (skin derivative)
Traits 4, 5, 12, 18 involve skin glands
All male sex traits are endocrinological; 13 is basically genetico-
   endocrinological.

Stage II. Testes, penis increase in size; scrotal skin furrowed, begins to darken; lightly pigmented downy ("silky") pubic hairs appear (12 ± 1).

Stage III. Penis length increases: downy pubic hairs give way to straight, coarse, pigmented terminal hair (13 ± 1).

Stage IV. Testes, penis increase in size (latter in both length and circumference); scrotal skin darker; pubic hair curly, semi-adult in pattern but smaller area (14 ± 1).

Stage V. Genitals and pubic hair pattern adult (15 ± 1, and on).

In Figure 39, from Tanner, is a schema of pubescent changes in the boy. The age period covered is 8–17 years. The height spurt has, on the average, its apex at about 14 years, but it may begin any time between 10½ and 16 years, end any time between 13½ and 17½ years. Note that the apex of the strength spurt is at the end of the height spurt, i.e., the boy is big *before* he is strong. Penis growth may begin any time between 10½ and 14½ years,

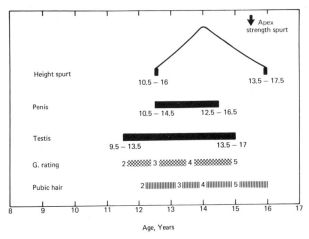

FIG. 39. Scheme of Sequence of Events in Adolescent Boys.

stop any time between 12½ and 16½ years. Similarly, testes growth may begin between 9½ and 13½ years, end between 13½ and 17 years. G. and pubic hair ratings based upon genital development and pubic hair pattern range, respectively, from 11½ to 15 years and from 12 to 16 years. Stages II to V are described in the text tabulation preceding the discussion of Figure 39.

Voice change in the boy occurs over a period of about one and a half years, from the first "break" to the final deeper tones. It is more highly correlated with skeletal age than with chronological age. According to general opinion the boy's voice falls a whole octave in its lower limit, about a sixth of an octave in its upper limit.

Changes in *head-hair* pattern for both boys and girls are seen in Figure 40. The immature forehead hair line in boys and in girls and women, is bowlike, convex upward as in A, B, C (this for whites; the Negro forehead

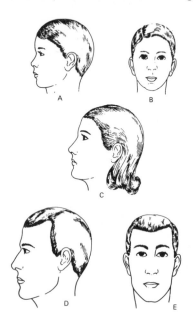

FIG. 40. Age-Changes in Hair Line Patterns in Boys and Girls.

hair line is not curved, but is horizontally straight). In mature white males, as in D and E, there are right and left fronto-temporal recessions, the *calvities frontalis adolescentium.* In males destined to become bald this fronto-temporal recession will move up, back, and toward the mid-line, resulting in an ever-increasing "high fore-head."

It is said that *muscle energy* doubles between the ages of ten and sixteen, as compared to the prepubertal boy. This is available energy—how closely it is related to muscular strength is not clear. At the completion of all the growth changes of adolescence, boys do have a larger muscle-mass and are able to develop more muscle force per gm of muscle. In middle and late adolescence the heart and lungs are large relative to total body size: more oxygen is carried in the blood and there is a greater capacity to neutralize the chemical products of muscular function, both in "resting" and functional use (exercise).

Events of Puberty: Girl

In the girl the major sex-changes revolve around breast development, body contouring (lateral "spread" of the hips, fat pads over hips, on abdomen, and over buttocks), genital growth (major and minor labia and vaginal tissues), body hair development (pubic and axillary), voice change, and "womanliness" in appearance and manner. As for the males, I offer here a "flow chart," listing a dozen female sex characteristics which are reasonably in sequence (p. 110). I must repeat that order and time (years are in parenthesis) are only average values. Time and order both vary, and may vary independently.

Shortly after the onset of the height spurt the bi-iliac (pelvic crest) or hip breadth begins to increase. At about the same time (some authorities put it first) the breast begins to "bud."

Shortly after the beginning of the height spurt, which is about two years earlier than in boys, girls begin to present the onset of secondary sex traits, mainly in bodily

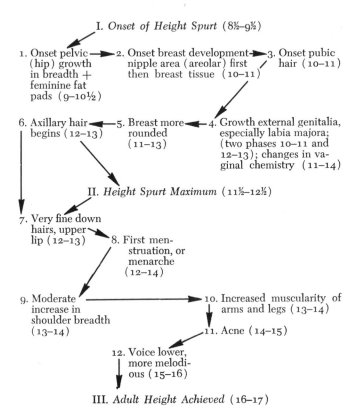

I. *Onset of Height Spurt* (8½–9½)

1. Onset pelvic → 2. Onset breast development → 3. Onset pubic
   (hip) growth   nipple area (areolar) first   hair (10–11)
   in breadth +   then breast tissue (10–11)
   feminine fat
   pads (9–10½)

6. Axillary hair ← 5. Breast more ← 4. Growth external genitalia,
   begins (12–13)   rounded   especially labia majora;
                      (11–13)   (two phases 10–11 and
                                           12–13); changes in va-
                                           ginal chemistry (11–14)

II. *Height Spurt Maximum* (11½–12½)

7. Very fine down
   hairs, upper
   lip (12–13)   8. First men-
                       struation, or
                       menarche
                       (12–14)

9. Moderate ──────────────→ 10. Increased muscularity of
   increase in   arms and legs (13–14)
   shoulder breadth
   (13–14)   11. Acne (14–15)

               12. Voice lower,
                   more melodi-
                   ous (15–16)

III. *Adult Height Achieved* (16–17)

Grouping
Traits 1, 2, 4, 5, 9, 10, 12 are morphological (structural)
Traits 3, 6, 7 are body hair (skin derivative)
Trait 11 involves skin glands
All female sex traits are endocrinological; 8 is more directly so.

contouring, i.e., increase in hip breadth and budding of
the breasts. Then, before the maximum expression of the
height spurt, changes in the genitalia occur, in two main
phases, about a year apart; the vaginal changes are concerned with cellular changes that lead to increased
glycogen content.

In a varying relation to time of maximum height
growth there occurs the *menarche* or the onset of men-

struation. After this time the changes that occur are largely non-sexual, i.e., they relate essentially to bodily contouring and voice changes. Finally, at sixteen and a quarter years, or later, adult height is achieved and womanhood has fully flowered.

In a summary form for girls, as was outlined for boys, we may recognize a number of stages in breast development. There are, indeed, two major categories, the first relating to the areolae (the pigmented area around the nipple), the second relating to the total configuration of the breast.

Areolar Stages, according to Garn, are as follows:

I. "Bud": papilla is embedded but the areolar area is slightly elevated.
II. "Mound": papilla still embedded, but areolar area is conically elevated.
III. "Mature": papilla is elevated, but in contrast the areolar area seems less conical.

Breast Stages are generally classified as follows:

I. Prepubertal: papilla present but no elevation whatsoever.
II. Onset: areolar elevation and slight mounding of breast tissue ($10\frac{1}{2} \pm 1$)
III. Mounded: breast swells to small mound (11 ± 1)
IV. Mature: breast is hemispherical; no further growth-oriented developmental changes ($12\frac{1}{2}-13\frac{1}{2} \pm 1$)

The development of *pubic hair* in the girl is classified into five stages, as follows:

I. Infantile: no pigmented hairs
II. Onset: sparse, pigmented hairs appear, principally on the labia majora; the hairs are straight to slightly curled and are moderately coarse. ($11-12 \pm 1$).
III. Intermediate: hair becomes curlier and spreads to the mons (the swelling on the lower abdomen at the top level of the pubic bones) ($12-13 \pm 1$).

iv. Subadult: continuation of III, but spread to inner aspect of the adjacent thighs (13 ± 1).

v. Adult: hair tightly curled; upper level horizontal to give a characteristically feminine triangular distribution (14 ± 1).

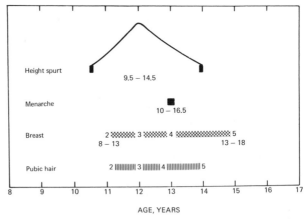

FIG. 41. Scheme of Sequence of Events in Adolescent Girls.

In Figure 41 Tanner offers a schema of pubescent changes in the girl. The age period covered is 8–17 years. The height spurt has its peak at 12 years, with a begin-end range of 10½–14 years. Menarche may occur, on the average, any time between 10 and 16½ years. Breast development begins its Stage II between 8 and 13 years and achieves definitive adult form (Stage V) by 13–18 years. Pubic hair begins Stage II at 11 years, achieves Stage V by 14 years. (For breast and pubic hair stages see the text.)

The voice change in the girl, from a rather shrill, thin sound to a "richer," fuller, more melodious tone, takes about a year and a half for complete transition. The lower level falls about one third of an octave, while the upper level rises about a third to a half of an octave.

In the listing of the time-sequence of sex traits in the girl the onset of menstruation (the menarche) was given as 12–14 years. This is, of course, only a central tendency.

The average age of the menarche in modern populations ranges from 12.2 years, reported for Cuban Negroes, to 18.8 years, reported for a New Guinea tribe, who are classed as Oceanic Negroids. Age at menarche is not earlier in one racial group or another, nor is it earlier in the tropics, later in temperate or Arctic climates. In a later discussion we shall note the factors affecting or modifying growth patterns, and we shall discover that rural vs. urban, better circumstanced social groups vs. the underprivileged, are potent factors making for group and individual variability.

Menarche

There has been noted a secular trend in statural increase. This same trend has operated to decrease or lower the average age of the menarche. In Norway in the 1840's the average age was seventeen years, one month, and in 1950 it was thirteen years, four months. In Germany in 1860 it was sixteen years, six months, and in 1935 it was thirteen years, five months. In Finland it was sixteen years, six months in 1860, and in 1940 it was fourteen years, and two months. In Sweden the average was fifteen years, seven months in 1890, and fourteen years, three months in 1940. The figures for Great Britain show a social class difference; the 1820 average for Manchester working women was fifteen years, eight months, for Manchester "educated ladies" it was fourteen years, seven months; in 1960 the average English girl had the menarche at thirteen years, three months. In the United States the average in 1905 was fourteen years, three months and in 1955 it was twelve years, nine months. The data for Poland show an urban-rural contrast: in Warsaw in 1875 the average was fifteen years, and in 1963 it was thirteen years; in the rural areas the average was seventeen years, three months in 1890, and fourteen years, nine months in 1955.

In seventy-six healthy California girls the length of the menstrual cycle ranged from 11 to 144 days, averaged

30.4 days, with the majority between 18 to 42 days. The duration of the menstrual period was 4.6 days, with a range of three to seven days.

There is an "adolescent sterility period" in girls, after the onset of the menarche, in the thirteenth to sixteenth year, an average of three years. Authors vary in their estimates of the duration of this sterility period from one to three "or more" years. Nubility thus is separated from menarche—whenever the menarche may occur—by about three years.

How much does a girl grow after the menarche? Does the timing of first menstruation permit the prediction of adult stature? These questions can be answered only approximately. On the average post-menarcheal growth is 2½–3″ (6.25–7.50 cm.), with a range of about 1″–7″. This range is a reflection of the fact that the girl who has the menarche early has it nearer the peak of her height-spurt, hence has more height growth left, as it were. Conversely, the girl who has the menarche late has it well after the peak of her height spurt, i.e., on the velocity curve for height growth she is well along in the terminal, decelerating phase. I have had many mothers of children at my Growth Center tell me, "I started to menstruate at eleven years or at twelve, when I was quite short—in a few years I became as tall as I am now," or "well, I did not menstruate until fifteen years and I was about the tallest girl among my friends—after that I slowed down."

Early-Late Maturation

The early-late dichotomy in sexual maturation occurs in both boys and girls: there are early boys, early girls, and late boys, and late girls—but regardless of category, the girls are at least two years ahead of the boys. Indeed, one might go so far as to say that earliness is female, lateness is male. Early sexual maturity is accompanied by an advanced skeletal age compared to chronological age.

Greulich (1942) reported on a study of primary and secondary sex changes in California boys. They were classified according to degree of advancement into five maturity categories. In boys age fifteen years, classed from least to most mature Groups I-II had an S.A. of 13.7 years, III of 14.2 years, IV of 14.9 years, V of 16.3 years. All were fifteen years old chronologically, but their growth age ranged from 13.7–16.3 years, a difference of 2.6 years.

Girls who achieve the menarche early are taller and heavier and are advanced in biological age. This is shown in Figures 42–44. These figures are based on the longitudinal study of Cleveland girls. Figures 42–43 show that

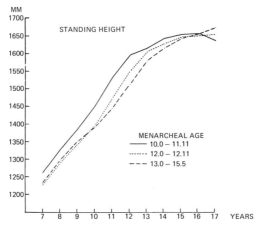

FIG. 42. Early-Late Menarche and Height, Age 7–17 Years.

from seven years of age and on girls with an early menarche are taller and heavier, respectively. However, at age sixteen years the "lates" catch up, more in height than in weight. Figure 44 shows that the early-maturing girl is advanced in biological age from seven to seventeen years and here there is *no* catch-up.

I present, in summary, a tabulation which depicts the total growth picture in the early vs. late boy and girl:

	EARLY		LATE	
Trait	*Boy*	*Girl*	*Boy*	*Girl*
1. Height as child	Tall	Tall	Short	Short
2. Weight as child	Stockier, heavier	Rounded, heavier	Slender, lighter	Slender, lighter
3. Period max. growth	Early	Early	Late	Late
4. Velocity of growth	Fast, for shorter period	Fast, for shorter period	Slow, for longer period	Slow, for longer period
5. Growth after sexual maturity achieved	Moderate to marked	Moderate to marked	Slight to moderate	Slight to moderate
6. Biological age (S.A.)	Advanced	Advanced	Retarded	Retarded
7. Adult body configuration	15–16 years	14–15 years	17–18 years (+)	15–16 years (+)
8. Physiological stability	Slight increase	No change	Slight increase	No change

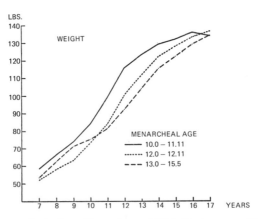

FIG. 43. Early-Late Menarche and Weight, Age 7–17 Years.

Adolescence

The adolescent boy and girl must relate to his or her total world, somewhat as schematized below:

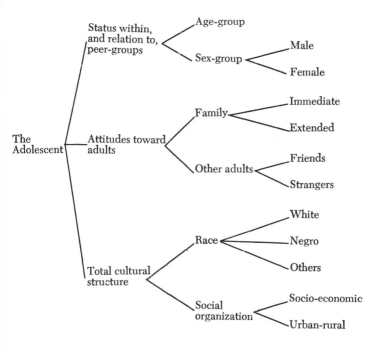

The age-group relationship has "two strikes against it," for there is involved the maturation age-chronological age and the sexual dichotomies. Both boys and girls are subject to the accelerated-laggard problem; for the "more mature" boys and girls often disassociate themselves from the "less mature." There is, further, the problem of the generalized biological priority of the girl who, suddenly on the threshold of womanliness, rejects yesterday's boy who is still a boy today.

The sex-grouping which in childhood is boy-boy, girl-girl, suddenly becomes boy-girl for both. Here, then, are all the problems of sex-realization for self and an awakened awareness in the boy of sexuality in the girl, and vice versa. The same early-late dichotomy probably holds here, too.

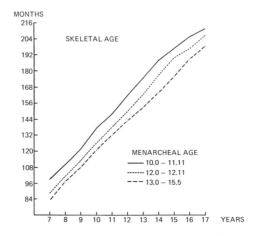

FIG. 44. Early-Late Menarche and Skeletal Age, Age 7–17 Years.

The attitude toward adults involves varying degrees of the so-called "generation gap." The adolescent's role in his own family (immediate) and to all of his relatives (extended) and to other adults (friends of the family, own friends, peer's families, teachers, and total strangers), is part of the entire reaction to "The Establishment."

The Establishment, of course, ramifies into the total cultural complex, with its almost hopeless entanglements of racial, class, and city-country attitudes and competitions. Here the adolescent comes to grips with "where the action is," and his part in it, now, and in the later years of his adult life.

In 1932 Todd wrote, almost prophetically, as follows:

> It is our business to see that these rapidly maturing boys and girls, who are still in half-lights and darkness, emerge quietly, simply, naturally, as themselves, and that they be not violently thrust into glories or terrors which they cannot understand.

In the nearly forty years that have passed since these words were written, changing socio-racial relations have made for a radically changed world; the "glories" have dimmed, the "terrors" have been re-focused. The adoles-

cent today is *self*-conscious far less with respect to biologi-
cal-self than with reference to social-self, at community,
national, and international levels. Events of today have in
a sense added to the sensitivities, frustrations, resent-
ments, emotional intensities, and rebellions that have always accompanied the childhood-to-adulthood, immatur-
ity-to-maturity, transition.

The sexual world, the socio-economic world, the politi-
cal world, are today more real to the adolescent than ever
before—not externally real, but internally, for he feels and
thinks of the problems, their handling, their solution, as
being of *his immediate concern*. He is the Don Quixote
who must tilt at the Establishment windmill: he, now,
with positive action!

All that is well, and I think it is good. But in this chapter I shall comment only upon the adolescent's sexual
world. The problems are absolute, for the adolescent feels
that his objective approach is the only one: sex is there, so
accept it in the sense of "doing the natural thing." The
problems are also relative, for whether the adolescent
likes it or not—or even realizes it—he can't tackle sex along
a united front, i.e., all adolescents equally able, or ready,
to cope with it. Biology still sets some of the ground-rules,
for the nature and degree of reaction and/or participation
is dependent upon an "earliness" or "lateness" grouping.

Sex Education

I sincerely feel that vastly better sex education is the
answer to the adolescent's question, "What *shall* I do
about sex?" The answer is not in the home. With all due
respect, the average parent is simply not competent to
teach sex at much better than a birds-and-bees "facts of
life" level.

The answer is to be found in programs of school education, which raises a certain number of problems:

1) Who shall teach? Not a "physical ed." coach, or in
a course of "Biology." It should be established as a separate course, in charge of a physician and a psychologist,

working in tandem. It should be given via the seminar method with a free question-and-answer situation at all times.

2) At what age should the instruction start? I would set about nine years as the best age. This is, in about ninety per cent of cases, the prepubertal time; the stage is set to give a prologue to the drama of sex. In most children puberty is imminent and they should have prepreparation. The average nine-year-old boy or girl has the mental equipment to understand, and many, via TV, magazine articles, and pictures, have experiential awareness.*

3) Should boys and girls be taught together? This is loaded with pros and cons. The pros (with whom I include myself) argue that sex will soon enough be shared experience, so why not share knowledge about sex together? The cons argue that embarrassment will hinder free and frank discussion. (But why assume embarrassment?) I take my stand for togetherness. I add, also, that I see no reason why a male physician should talk to the boys separately, a female physician to the girls separately. The sex of the instructor need not militate against pooling the sexes for sex instruction.

4) What should be taught? The biology of sex, certainly, along with some idea of sequence and time (age) of the various aspects of sexual maturation. The role of sex in male-female relationships, with emphasis upon marriage as a generally accepted sexual relationship. This need not rest upon various forms and/or systems of re-

*My selection of nine years as a beginning age is biased, I must admit, in a biological direction. I am swayed by growth-timing, for age nine is really at a major transition age, from mid to late childhood, from slower growth to a heightened tempo, from a relatively static growth phase to one of great and dynamic changes. At age nine adult proportions, i.e., adult body construct, are foreshadowed—"manliness" and "womanliness" are incipient. Then, too, peer-grouping has set the stage for the male-female dichotomy just ahead.

ligious sanction, but rather a family-type situation as nuclear to a more satisfactory adjustment.

5) What about other aspects of sex: premarital relations, contraception, homosexuality? With respect to the problem of premarital relations the situation is best handled on a psychological than on a purely medical or religio-moralistic basis. Essentially, the hazards of a psychologically unsatisfactory emotional response and relationship are the chief points to be stressed. Certainly the risk of disease and pregnancy should be stressed. However, sole appeal on the basis of "It isn't right," or "Wait until you get married," or "It is a sin," are apt to be met with rejection and disdain. As for contraceptive practices, certainly they should be taught. The right to have children—almost, indeed, the right to be born—is part of human free will. The decision must be stressed as an individual human right. The problems of homosexuality should be frankly discussed. The news media are full of stories of relaxed laws regarding homosexual behavior, the movies portray it, jokes about it are common, so meet the problem objectively with discussion of its nature and its effects upon individuals and upon the community.

VIII

ROLES OF NUTRITION AND
ENVIRONMENT IN GROWTH

The Problems of Nutrition

I'll bet against any odds that an Old Stone Age Cave-
woman said something like this to her son, "now, Snag-
tooth, I want you to eat that Cavebear meat. It's good for
you. I cooked it over those black stones that burn so well.
And eat those wild herbs and vegetables. And drink that
mare's milk. You want to grow up big and strong like
your father, The One Who Sees Far, the mighty hunter,
don't you?" I am just as willing to bet that from earliest
times Man knew, in principle, that "we are what we eat!"

Plato (ca. 428–348 B.C.) said:

> Meats and drinks come in from without, and are compre-
> hended in the body . . . the frame of the body gets the
> better of them . . . and so the animal grows great, being
> nourished by a multitude of similar particles.

At about the same time Aristotle (ca. 384–322 B.C.),
observed:

> For everywhere the nutriment may be divided into two
> kinds; the first and the second, the former is "nutritious,"
> being that which gives its essence both to the whole and to
> the parts; the latter is concerned with growth, that which
> causes quantitative increase.

On the day you read this, three out of every four people in the world will go to bed hungry. Over three hundred million growing children in the developing countries of the world, *and* also in the urban areas of industrialized countries, are in grave danger from under- or malnutrition. They will make the grade for six months to a year or so, on mother's milk, then they'll falter, so that in a few years their height and weight will be only at the 10th-15th percentile. Many will die before they are four years old; their mortality rate between one and four years will be twenty to forty times greater than in North America and most of the countries in Europe.

The picture is all too common in "the misery spots" of the world. Most serious (in addition to caloric deficiency) is the protein deficit: the total protein intake will be less than one fourth of American standards, and animal protein less than one tenth. Not only will size be inhibited, the growth of the tissue mass may even be reversed; bones will be thin, muscles wasted, and behavioral development will be retarded and even, in some respects, permanently stultified. The total child, under such conditions, can only be a warped, twisted, poorly responsive organism, whose potential role as an adult must reflect the poor nutritional soil in which he was nurtured. Never more true is the saying, "As the twig is bent. . . ."

If I were to attempt to draw up a scheme or a community blueprint of factors contributing to nutritional inadequacy I should have to foray into a total socio-cultural analysis: levels of technological development plus the buying power to take advantage of technological tools; purchasing levels of income within the population concerned; likewise, levels of education so that cultural advances may be incorporated within the total group; available foodstuffs, in variety and in amount; community and family sanitation; availability of medical and dental care; marriage-patterns, in terms of inbreeding and of outbreeding (the former may intensify unfavorable or dysgenic biological and behavioral patterns). . . . I could go on and on, but I would only belabor the point: that the *total environment* of the growing child is involved. Nutrition is not an all-or-none factor; rather it is a one-of-many factor, albeit a very important factor. There is another thing about such a "blueprint," viz., with a few modifications it applies to the densely crowded urban areas the world over; (the "black ghettos" of the United States, the squalid "shack-towns" of many large cities in Europe, Africa, Asia). Starvation has little set geography, it has no politics, it has no national bounds; it has only the inequalities, the inequities, of man's socio-cultural systems, only the incredible ineptitudes of lack of long-term thinking and planning. When stripped to essentials, what is a "ghetto" or a "shack-town" but a village pattern grafted into an urban construct? Here in the United States our nuclei of misery in big cities are outmoded socio-economic units that have festered into disfiguring excrescences.

General Requirements

The nutritional requirements for good, well-balanced growth are extremely complex and can only be sketchily presented. The growing child needs, we are told, a total minimum balance about as follows: 1) twenty-three amino acids; 2) one source of glucose (carbohydrate); 3) one fat (an unsaturated fatty acid called linoleic acid); 4) at least five vitamins (A, B complex, C, D, K); 5) eleven inorganic elements (calcium, chlorine, copper, iodine, iron, magnesium, manganese, phosphorus, potassium, sodium, sulphur).

The above complex may be regrouped into five major kinds of chemicals we need for a total, well-balanced diet.

1. Vitamins: the catalysts (the chemical "workhorses") to speed the synthesis of new compounds
2. Minerals (Vitamins and minerals are ready for immediate use)
3. Proteins (which split into twenty-three amino acids)

4. Carbohydrate, as simple sugars for energy
5. Fats to give fatty acids plus glycerol.

If any sort of priority be given to any one of the above five kinds of chemicals it must go to No. 3, the proteins.

Structurally proteins are the basic components of skin, hair, muscle, blood vessels, and internal organs. Functionally they yield enzymes, hemoglobin, and some hormones, e.g., insulin. In the growth-period of birth-twenty years, the body snythesizes 500–1000 lbs of protein, half of which replaces worn-out or damaged cells. At twenty years the total body protein weighs twenty to forty lbs, and forms eighty per cent of the non-water weight of muscle, ninety per cent of the non-water weight of blood, and thirty-five per cent of the dry weight of bone.

It is scant wonder, therefore, that nutritionists point out that a difference of only ten calories per day per kilogram of body weight, and a few milligrams of protein per day per kilogram of body weight, make the difference between successful or failing growth. The balance is disconcertingly fine!

Prenatal Growth and Nutrition

The human fetus gains weight more slowly than most other mammals. At twenty-six weeks the weight averages 900 gm, which equals a rate of 5.0 gm per day. In the next four weeks, for a newborn who will weigh 3500 gm, the gain averages 20 gm per day, and after that (to birth) the average is 35 gm per day. Here, according to Dean (1960), is a summary of daily gain *in utero*.

Age	Weight (gms.)	Protein (gms.)	Fat (gms.)	Calorie Value
0–182 days	7	0.7	0.05	3.5
182–210 days	29	3.5	2.0	34.0
210–238 days	36	5.0	5.5	66.0
238–278 days	45	5.0	10.0	114.0

Adequate and balanced nutrition starts at conception, and is specially important in the first three postconceptual months (first trimester). During this time the quantity of food intake need not be increased; after that, in the second and third trimesters, it should be. The pregnant female should increase her daily protein intake to 1.5 gm per kg of body weight. Calcium and phosphorous should each be increased to 1.5 gm per kg body weight daily; iron intake should correspondingly go up to 15 mg, iodine to 0.15–0.30 mg. In the vitamins, D should go to a daily 400 I.U. (International Units), A to a daily 6000 I.U., ascorbic acid to a daily 100 mg, and the B complex should also be increased (determined on an individual basis). Such a prenatal maternal intake will fit in with an allowable maternal gain of twenty lbs (9 kg).

The relation of maternal diet to the physical condition of the newborn is summarized by Stuart (1941) of Harvard as follows:

Condition of Infant	Maternal Diet			
	Superior	Good	Fair	Poor(est.)
Good to Excellent (31)	42%	52%	3%	3%
Fair (149)	6%	44.5%	44.5%	5%
Poor to Very Poor (36)	3%	6%	25%	66%

(Nos. in parentheses = size of sample in each category)

In 180 of the 216 newborn who were in Excellent to Fair condition the maternal diet was Superior to Good.

At birth *bone development* was rated for both protein and calcium intake on a five-point scale (excellent, good, fair, poor, very poor). For protein intake, in the Excellent group fifty-seven per cent of the newborn were advanced, twenty-nine per cent average, fourteen per cent retarded, while in the Very Poor group the figures were zero per cent, twenty-nine per cent and seventy-one per cent, respectively. For calcium intake the Excellent group showed thirty-two per cent advanced, forty-five per cent average, twenty-three per cent retarded, while the Very Poor group showed six per cent, thirty per cent, sixty-four per cent, respectively.

At birth *dental development* was evaluated on the same basis as for bones. For protein intake the Excellent group showed thirty-seven per cent advanced, forty-seven per cent average, sixteen per cent retarded, while the Very Poor group showed zero per cent, twenty-nine per cent, seventy-one per cent, respectively. For calcium intake the Excellent group showed twenty-eight per cent advanced, forty-eight per cent average, twenty-four per cent retarded, while the Very Poor group showed ten per cent, twenty-eight per cent, sixty-two per cent, respectively.

Bone and tooth maturation are both adversely affected by a poor prenatal maternal diet, as at least measured by protein and calcium intake. Of the two, protein deficiency hits a bit harder. A good start for a human life begins, apart from heredity, with a good prenatal maternal nutrition.

Postnatal Growth and Nutrition

Early in this chapter I listed the *"General Requirements"* of nutritive intake. Now let us look at the *Specific Requirements* for the birth-twenty year growth period. The data to be presented are from two major sources: the National Research Council of the U.S., and Watson and Lowrey (1967). In terms of total *caloric* need the latter authors suggest that growth needs to be broken down into five basic categories: 1) basal metabolism; 2) specific dynamic action of organs and/or systems; 3) loss via excretion; 4) activity demands; 5) demands of growth per se. The following tabulation is from Table 47 of Watson and Lowrey, and is based on cal/kg (calories per kilogram of body weight).

Need/age	8 wks.	10 mos.	4 yrs.	Adult
Basal	55	55	40	25
S.D.A.	7	7	6	—
Excreta	11	10	8	47±
Activity*	17	20	25±	6
Growth	20	12	8–10	6
Totals	110	104	87–89±	10±

*The activity needs will be certainly stepped-up during the surge of growth at puberty and adolescence, especially among boys.

Protein need (gm/kg) (grams per kilogram of body weight) is four in infancy, three at five years, two at 10 years, and one at 15 years and as adult. *Water* intake (cc/kg) (centimeters per kilogram of body weight) is, respectively, 150, 100, 75, and levels at 50.

The daily *vitamin* requirements of the growing child may be summarized, after Watson and Lowrey, in the following fashion: vitamin A is necessary for good vision and tissue health; in terms of International Units (I.U.) amount ranges from 2,000 I.U. in infancy, 3,000 I.U. at five years, and 4,000 I.U. at ten years; vitamin D is necessary for calcium and phosphorus metabolism (bones and teeth); up to ten years 400–800 I.U. is sufficient; vitamin C is necessary for the metabolism of amino acids and for cellular and tissue well-being; needed are 30 mg, 50 mg, and 70 mg in infancy, at 5:0, and at 10:0, respectively; vitamin K is necessary for blood-clotting, with intake amounts not definite; niacin aids in cellular oxidation; intake is 0.6 mg, 1.2 mg, and 1.8 mg, for infancy, 5:0, and 10:0, respectively; riboflavin aids in cellular respiration; intake is 0.6 mg, 1.2 mg, and 1.8 mg, for infancy, 5.0, and 10:0, respectively, thiamine is necessary to the metabolism of pyruvic acid; intake is 0.4 mg, 0.8 mg, and 1.2 mg for infancy, 5.0, and 10:0, respectively.

Foods containing these vitamins include the following as basic sources: milk (A, niacin, riboflavin, thiamine); eggs (A, riboflavin, thiamine); meats (A and niacin in beef, riboflavin and thiamine in pork); liver (A, D in fish oils, niacin, riboflavin); citrus fruits (C); leafy vegetables (A, K); fruits other than citrus (riboflavin); cereals (thiamine); soy beans, rice (K)

The foregoing nutritional requirements are based on recent and current researches. However, long before such precise information was available the effects of varying ethnic diets had been observed and conclusions as to the importance of adequate and balanced diets in growth had been inferred.

An early breakthrough on the effect of nutrition on postnatal growth was that achieved in the early 1900's by McCarrison, an English nutritionist. Col. McCarrison was in the Army Medical Corps, and while on duty in India was struck by differences in adult size among the tribes and castes. In Central India he noted two groups, who lived side-by-side, the Rajputs and the Chuhras, who, said the anthropologists, were racially identical. Yet the Rajputs were six-footers, the Chuhras below even average statures; also the former were high-caste, the latter among the low-caste "untouchables." The Rajputs had good to very good living conditions, including food intake; the Chuhras were underprivileged, and, indeed, their living area was classed among the "misery spots" of India. The conclusion seemed obvious: since the two populations were genetically (racially) alike, their size differences (which represented the summations of growth) must be due not alone to their total living conditions, but to the latter group's very poor nutrition.

A few years later McCarrison demonstrated this experimentally. He selected two contrasting Indian diets: 1) *Sikh,* meat, vegetables, grain, milk; 2) *Madrassi,* vegetables, rice, coffee, betel nuts. Laboratory animals reared on the Sikh diet were by far larger, better developed age-wise, and healthier.

What has often been referred to as a "classic" study is that of Mann (1926), who observed three hundred fifty institutionalized English school-age boys for two years. To the control basic middle-class institution diet he added various dietary supplements, noting height and weight gains, basically the latter as the more significant. The control group gained 3.85 lbs in one year. The experimental group, listed by the dietary supplements, gained as follows: casein, 4.01 lbs (+4.2%, compared to control); sugar, 4.93 lbs (+28.1%); margarine, 5.21 lbs (+35.3%); watercress, 5.40 lbs (+40.3%); butter, 6.30 lbs (+63.6%); milk, 6.98 lbs (+81.3%).

In the United States, a dozen years later, Roberts and her associates firmly demonstrated the growth-promoting merit of a protein-enriched food intake. Again, the diet of institutionalized children was used as a control. A dietary supplement was set up as one pint of milk daily, plus five eggs per week, plus three ounces of cheese per week, plus ten ounces of ice cream per week. In one year the children on the basic diet gained, for age, only 61 per cent of expected weight and 80 per cent of expected height. The supplemented group gained one hundred forty per cent and one hundred two, respectively. Most importantly, however, the latter group, in the next few years (although no longer on the buffered diet), gained height and weight equal to, or a bit above, the average values of normative "standards."

There is no use in citing further evidence: study after study could be quoted that an adequate (in calories) and a balanced diet (in protein, minerals, vitamins) is growth-promoting. We most often measure good nutrition by weight gain, but the real measure is well-being, which depends less on the adequacy of energy-producing foods than on the balanced protective foods. It is these which ensure the buoyancy of good and resilient health.

Nutrition and Maturation

It is not enough to speak of *size* alone—weight, height, possibly other bodily dimensions—with respect to the nutritive factor. There is an equally important part of the picture, viz., *maturation,* which is an indication of general bodily development. This can be measured in terms of the skeletal age as assessed at least in the hand-wrist X-ray film, or additionally in X-ray films of elbow, knee, and foot.

It is an intriguing point to make that, while in our Congress we talk about malnutrition in "tens of thousands of American children" we have little or no really good controlled serial growth data on any sample of these "thousands." We have to go to Central America, Africa, or Asia Minor/Asia for illustrative material—and much of that focuses on weight, with height as an afterthought, and maturation too often an also-ran. In a Turkish study, four groups of school children were set up, going from moderate (I) to very severe malnutrition (IV). All had X-ray films of hand and wrist. An American standard of film assessment was used, which may have introduced a slight and constant bias, i.e., American standard "higher" than for other groups. At all events here are the results: in Group I the skeletal age (S.A.) averaged 88.75% of the chronological age (C.A.); in Group II the S.A. averaged 71.22% of the C.A.; in Group III the S.A. averaged 53.86% of the C.A.; in Group IV the S.A. averaged 39.95% of the C.A.

There can be no doubt that malnutrition and retarded maturation go together, and that the severer the one, the more marked the other. This relatively simple statement is not enough: it is not size alone, or maturation alone, that is affected in a retardant direction, but it is likely that *all* bodily systems are retarded or deviated in their development. Moreover, the younger the child the more widespread or diffused the effects of very severe malnutrition, especially, as has been said, if protein insufficiency is involved.

It is not stretching a point to say that protein-calorie deficiency during growth is literally a *bone disease*. The bone tends to grow at the expense of its own total bone volume. The result is a greatly reduced cortex (outer structure) compared to medulla (inner marrow cavity), i.e., long, thin-shelled, relatively fragile long bones. Over and beyond this, the hand and foot bones in such deficiency show many more anomalous centers of ossification, and the growing shafts of the long-bones many more "scars of arrested growth." In even finer detail the texture of the bones (the trabeculation or inter-lacing of bone fibers as seen in the X-ray films) changes, essentially in a demineralized or osteoporotic direction.

Sexual maturation is part of the nutrition picture, as might be expected. In girls menarche is delayed under conditions of malnutrition, normally timed or even advanced under optimum conditions of nutrition. Indeed, one of the major reasons adduced for the secular decrease in menarcheal age is the improved nutrition of Occidental civilization in general.

If we group size, bone maturation age, bone structure, and sexual maturation age at this point then the nutrition problem takes on a formidable complexity. This combination of retardations and structural inadequacies suggests a general and probably deep-seated involvement. The answer is, "yes, but the total mechanism is not clear." One thing *is* reasonably clear, namely that there is probably a hormonal involvement: it seems logical to assume that one of the effects of severe malnutrition is to cause a *functional* anterior lobe hypopituitarism. There is no real pathology involved—the anterior pituitary just doesn't function as well as it should, and it does not secrete the necessary amounts of the growth and sex-stimulating hormones that it should. It just slows down!

The World Nutrition Problem

Severe malnutrition, involving both calorie and protein deficiency, is a world problem, and, since the United States is committed to the economic aid of under-developed and developing countries, it is an American problem, too. In many areas of the world half of the children in low-income brackets die before five years of age. A significant number of these die of malnutrition, usually after weaning. In the United States and Europe the mortality rate between one and four years of age is 1:1000; in many underdeveloped areas it ranges from 10:1000 to 45:1000.

Protein and calorie deficiency in their severest growth-failure forms give rise to *kwashiorkor* and *marasmus*. The former basically involves protein deficiency and hits hardest between two and three years of age. In one area of Africa of 1,141 children with kwashiorkor, eighty-six per cent died by age three years. The latter involves protein + calorie deficiency and hits hardest in the first year of life. In Figure 45 is shown the world distribution of kwashiorkor, with Central and South America, Africa, and Asia

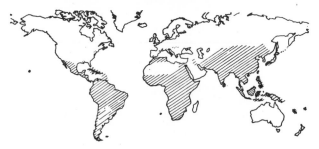

FIG. 45. Geographical Distribution of Kwashiorkor.

Minor and Southern Asia as focal areas. North America and Europe are not involved, but some of the urban ghettos in the United States are reputedly not far from it. There may be differences in degree, but hardly in basic kind.

Kwashiorkor and marasmus form a total spectrum of nutritional failure, but there are some differences between the two. The marasmic child is retarded in weight, height, and maturation, i.e., is a failure in both growth and development. He has very marked muscular atrophy, and an almost complete absence of subcutaneous fat.

The child with kwashiorkor is characterized by "pitting" edema and an apathetic, irritable manner. His muscle tone is poor. His skin shows "rashes" and peels in spots. His hair becomes brittle, falls out easily, and becomes depigmented (it has a "flag sign" [see Figure 46]

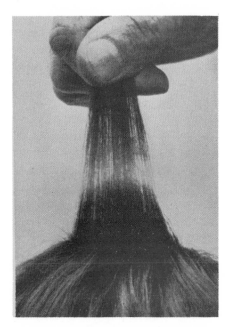

FIG. 46. The "Flag Sign" in the Head Hair of a Child with Kwashiorkor.

due to bands of color loss when the condition is severe). The appetite is poor and diarrhea is severe (often with undigested food). There are numerous biochemical changes in blood, liver, gut, muscles. The brain waves show low rhythmic activity. On the Gesell tests for psychomotor and behavioral development there is often severe retardation.

There is no escaping the fact that marasmus and kwashiorkor are still the diseases of the infants of the world born to the nutritionally most deprived. The effects of such extreme malnutrition are dramatically striking and have commanded a humanitarian response, yet the every-dayness of undernutrition throughout the world— including the United States—cannot be overlooked. Wherever there are marked differences in cultural levels from extremes of poverty to the comforts of the middle and upper classes, there are corresponding differences in amount and balance of nutritive intake that are reflected in growth and maturation. In times of total cultural upheaval the nutritional levels suffer accordingly.

As the aftermath of World War I, studies in Berlin, Stuttgart, Munich (the big cities showed the more drastic growth failure) revealed that in 1917–1918 the intake of protein, calories, and fat had been reduced by thirty-three per cent or more. There was a general growth retardation, more in weight than in height, more in boys than in girls, so marked that the secular gains of previous decades were wiped out. World War II showed much the same results, but in some countries it was more marked, especially in Nazi-occupied areas. The suppression of food intake in these countries was carefully, and even scientifically, planned: diets were sub-minimal with intake of calories, protein, calcium, and vitamins deliberately low. For these children an analysis of maturation was added to the height-weight parameters: not only were the school-age children small (an inch to an inch and a half shorter, ten pounds lighter) compared to prewar age and sex standards, but they were lagging a year or more in maturational progress. In Occupied France, for example, adolescent girls did not, in the late war years or early years after cessation of war, achieve the menarche until an average age of sixteen years.

Catch-up Growth

The nongenetic factors of malnutrition pose several questions: how intense or how long must be the damage to effect a growth slow-down? how lasting is this slow-down? will it really stultify growth, i.e., will it affect the growth potential of the child? what are the mechanisms involved in the slow-down? The last question may be answered, I think, in terms of a *stress* mechanism. There can be no doubt that mal- and/or undernutrition stress

the growing organism in terms of all biological parameters. The first thing one thinks of is a possible reaction
of the endocrine system: there may be a twofold effect,
i.e., a decrease in the pituitary growth hormone (anabolic
or growth-promoting), and an increase in adrenal cortisol
(anti-anabolic or growth-inhibiting). It has been suggested that in the metabolic disturbance of malnutrition
(and of illness) the child mobilizes the amino acids for
stress-combat rather than for bone growth.

It is worthy of note that in these nutritional insults it
is growth in size that is hit harder than maturational
progress. This is a very important fact, for if skeletal
maturation were markedly retarded then union of centers
of long-bone growth would be delayed, with a corresponding increase in the duration of growth-time. This is
not the case, for size must recover—if it *does* recover—
in only a little more time than in the healthy child. An
example may make this clearer: suppose that we have
two boys aged five years, each with a growth potential
of 68″; at age five years both are 45″ tall (23″ to go); one
of the boys is malnourished or is ill and registers an age-
standard loss of ¾″ and a maturation retardation of six
months; therefore this boy at age five years must "make
up" ¾″ in only six months more of growing time compared to the other boy who enjoys good food intake and
health.

The terms "make-up" and "catch-up" are the crux of
the recovery theme in growth retarded or inhibited by
poor nutrition or illness or any other variable. The problem is not a simple one: to be evaluated are degree and
kind of damage, its duration, timing in term of child's
age, treatment given, and so on. The basic principles of
the interrelation of these variables have been developed
by animal experiments in the 1910's and 1920's. The experimental animal was underfed in varying amounts, for
varying periods of time, at varying ages, and then put
back on an adequate or buffering diet; in some experi-

ments the off-again, on-again interplay was repeated several times. The effects of starvation on size and bone maturation were recorded and then the recovery effects of good nutrition. As a general rule there was more or less catch-up growth. The basic findings of the animal experiments may be applied to human growth and maturation.

In 1966 Graham, Cordono and their colleagues treated seventeen infants with severe malnutrition at 6–13 months, and a follow-up at 17–30 months. The body weight gain, for the respective periods, was 2.5 and 4.0 times the normal rate; head circumference similarly had a rate gain of 2.2 and 4.6 times the normal rate. With regard to body length those with a deficit of five per cent or less caught up, but those with a fifteen plus per cent deficit did not—they remained significantly short; those between five and fifteen per cent caught up at an accelerated rate.

The reasons for catch-up growth are complex and unclear. Restoration of hormonal balance has been mentioned and in very severe retardation this may well be a factor. Other suggestions focus upon the growth potential in the individual child, assuming, in principle, that the child has an inherent and presumably genetic path of growth; the concept of "path" has been called "channelization" or "canalization." The idea is something like this: via poor nutrition, or ill health, the child is, so to speak, detoured from his path in a slowed-up, size-inhibited direction. The recovery phase, via appropriate therapy, will once more put the child on the main road.

Nutrition and Behavior

It is now time to turn our attention to a problem that is at once difficult to measure and difficult to interpret. The problem may be stated, "Do the factors that retard or inhibit growth and maturation also retard or inhibit brain growth and behavioral development, including intellectual capacity?" Answers to this question come from both animal experiments and human studies.

A rat has eighty per cent of its brain growth by four weeks after birth, a pig in eight to ten weeks, but the rest of the body has achieved only twenty per cent of its adult values. In a child the brain weight is eighty per cent of its adult value by three years, but the rest of the body has only twenty per cent. Hence, a child takes three years to achieve, in terms of brain growth, what a rat does in four weeks, a pig in eight to ten weeks. In the infant experimental animals given diets severely deficient in proteins, there is central nervous system damage: brain waves diminish in rhythmic activity; in the brain-stem and in the spinal cord there are degenerative changes in several types of nerve cells. Even if the animals are given a high-protein diet for three months after deprivation, the clinical condition is improved but the central nervous system still shows damage at cell-level. These animals show behavioral changes, plus a lowered capacity to perform tests requiring *learning* based on multiple trials. In another study it was found that rats born of malnourished mothers showed behavioral changes when nursed by these mothers; they did much better with well-nourished foster-mothers.

When we turn to children we meet a much more complex situation. Insufficient food is certainly a factor. But add to that a total family situation, possibly involving alcoholism, rejection, poor sanitation, inadequate health care, poor educational and recreational facilities, illegitimacy, a "broken" home, lack of motivation due to repeated rebuffing, and so on. Who then may say which straw broke which camel's back?

It is necessary to cite only one or two examples of the nutrition-behavior relationship from studies carried on in Africa and Central and South America, where research and remedial care are doing a not-enough best. In Chile, fourteen children were diagnosed between one and five months of age as being marasmic. They were treated over a long time at a hospital, then seen in the out-patient department. Upon being discharged from the hospital the mother was given twenty liters of free milk per month for each child. From three to six years later the children were clinically all right and had achieved weight and height standards for age. But the head circumference and the I.Q. were both significantly less than for normal, healthy children, for age and for sex. Importantly, *language skill* was the most retarded. In Cape Town, in "apartheid" South Africa, a series of I.Q. tests carried out over a ten-year period on malnourished Bantu children showed consistently lower scores than for adequately nourished Bantu controls. The children were short, were underweight, had smaller brains (as deduced from head dimensions), had reduced rhythmic brain activity, and did very poorly in tests involving visual perception.

It might be argued that the I.Q. is: 1) inherently unreliable, and 2) not applicable to children of a different culture, but this is playing ostrich. The same tests show *within-group* differences, always sorting out the failures (malnourished) and the successful (well nourished). In the United States it has been shown that children who lag progressively in bodily growth and maturation lag progressively in learning behavior: 1) block-piling, an eye-hand neuromuscular test; 2) linguistic activities, as in naming objects or parts of own body; 3) visual-perceptive activities, such as a form-board. It is a fair generalization to say that the *entire learning process* is involved: negatively in the mal- or undernourished child, positively in the normal healthy child.

It is no wonder that Scrimshaw states that ". . . nutritional deficiency, if sufficiently early and severe, can have profound and permanent detrimental consequences for the learning and behavior of children." Or, "malnutrition can interact with infection, heredity, and social factors to bring about physical and mental impairment."

The past few pages point to us, here in the affluent United States society. Whether we like it or not, we have our own "misery spots," perhaps relatively in most instances, rather than absolutely. They are urban for the most part and they are predominantly among the American Negroes. *The problem is not racial,* except insofar as darker skins may have been targets—but *this is cultural.* We have our "Project Head Start," which starts at about four years of age. It is four years—nay, four years, nine months—too late. It should start prenatally, accelerate circumnatally, and guarantee each child—Negro and white—a Good Start for every day, week, month, year on the road of growth and development.

I cannot leave the discussion of nutrition without a few remarks upon the current American diet scene. These remarks, made by a leading nutritionist, are aimed equally at the growing child and at the adult.

According to Dr. Jean Mayer, formerly Presidential Advisor on Nutrition under President Johnson, Americans, young and old, do not eat right. Our diets, he says, are too rich in fats, too poor in other nutrients. For example, the per cent of fat in the diet has risen from twenty-five per cent in 1900 to more than forty per cent today (in some groups as high as fifty per cent). We are beset by "diet fads": a Harvard study showed that ninety-seven per cent of adolescent girls were on "some kind" of a diet, either to gain weight or to lose it or, hopefully, to redistribute it!

The answer? Fewer total calories, less fat, less sugar— a more balanced diet . . . *and more healthy exercise.* For whom the shoe fits let the dinner bell toll more softly, or less frequently!

The Total Environment: Social Structure

The word "environment" has so many definitions, means such different things to different people, that one almost hesitates to use it. Literally, the environment (in referring to growth) is everything that surrounds the child—it is the sum of all effects, and most often the effects are taken to be outer or external, as opposed to within or internal. The outer effects are referred to as *exogenous,* the inner as *endogenous;* the two are basic to the old question of "environment vs. heredity," respectively. *In utero* the total maternal organism is the environment. Postnatally, the whole outside world moves in, successively: the mother, both parents, siblings, if any. Parents and siblings form the nuclear family. Then come all relatives who comprise the extended family. Next, the neighborhood, the social classes, the total community, and so on. Included in the social structure is the family again, for the father, as wage-earner and "head of the family," has much to do with the socio-economic milieu in which the child is being reared. The immediate family, especially the mother, sets the emotional framework within which the child is nurtured and matures. Obviously, the total environment is the sum of both tangible and intangible impacts upon the growing child. Add to this the way in which the child internalizes the stimuli and the way in which the child reacts to them, then the entire environmentally influenced and/or modified growth pattern becomes complex indeed.

When one speaks of growth differences in children of different *socio-economic* levels one need hark back only to the discussion in the first half of this chapter, for food *is* related to the socio-economic system. Thus class income is most often scaled from professional men (physicians, dentists, lawyers, business executives and the academic world); the "white collar" employee group; and the "blue collar" labor group (skilled and unskilled). This is the customary hierarchy, from above down. Income is scaled at a certain optimum and above, to a certain average, and to a certain minimum. In these groupings the "food dollar" ranges from plentiful to an extremely stretched-out bare amount, going on into welfare ranks. Certainly nutrition is not the sole factor, but it *is* a basic one. Be that as it may the evidence of facilitated or inhibited child growth in an upper-lower social class dichotomy is a very real thing.

Stature and Maturation and Social Class

Studies in the United States have shown that boys in the upper classes average, age for age, three per cent taller and six per cent heavier. A German study revealed that a fifteen-year-old boy in the top social class was 4.3 cm (1.7″) taller than a like-aged boy in the lowest class. A study of some seventy-five hundred Glasgow (Scotland) boys aged nine years, showed those in the "highest occupational class" to be 2.11″ taller than nine-year-old boys in the lowest. In the United States, during the depression a study was made in 1933 of two school-age groups in a severely depressed industrial area; the groups were 1) those receiving free lunch and/or welfare funds, and 2) those whose parents could not qualify for civic aid. The children of group 1) were consistently two and a half to nine lbs. underweight for age compared to the children of group 2). In other words the children most in need of supplementary aid were receiving it.

A very thorough study in Switzerland went beyond height-weight growth in the children of four social classes: 1) unskilled labor; 2) semiskilled labor; 3) clerical; 4) professional, administrative, academic. The children of classes 3) and 4) were taller, heavier, had broader shoulders and hips, and greater arm and leg circumferences (upper arm, thigh, calf). While skinfold measurements and skin-fat-muscle-bone radiography were not taken, the greater limb circumferences almost certainly point to a greater subcutaneous fat layer. In groups 1) and 2) there were 2.57 children per family, and in groups 3) and 4) 2.17 children per family. Hence, family size, per se, was not a factor in this study.

It is all well and good to cite data as in the foregoing paragraphs, but on a chronological age basis the differences may be more apparent than real. It is very likely that two boys, both aged ten years by the calendar, one in an upper class, the other in a lower, may not be really comparable, especially if family-size differs radically, i.e., larger family in the lower-class child, smaller in the upper-class child. Studies of *growth-rate* have shown that the larger the family the slower the growth-rate. This is evident by the sixth year and continues thereafter, so that the adolescent growth spurt (betokening a maturational level) is also delayed. As a general rule, therefore, it may be accepted that in many children of the lower income brackets there may be a threefold reaction in the growth pattern: 1) smaller size; 2) slower rate; 3) retarded or inhibited maturation.

The Emotional Environment

The maternal role in growth of the child is basically important in all aspects of development. The whole realm of child care is involved. I shall here mention only two aspects, the one physical, the other emotional. On the physical side there is a significant and positive correlation between maternal size (weight, especially) and the weight of the newborn child. This correlation increases when the mother is over thirty years of age and when the child is third-born or later; the correlation is also slightly greater when the interval between births is two years or more.

When the child is grossly neglected by the mother—for whatever reason—there may develop the "Maternal Deprivation Syndrome," wherein the child is retarded in growth and maturation, and in severe cases may show a retarded motor and intellectual development. Patton and Gardner reported on the growth of five infants over an age span of thirteen to thirty-six months in a poor home situation: their height was forty-two per cent below the norm for age and sex; they were "extremely" underweight; their skeletal age was greatly retarded, and the long bones of arms and legs showed many "scars of arrested growth." Even after removal from the disastrous maternal environment they did not easily return to an acceptable personality structure and intellectual performance. The authors suggested a "block" in anabolic growth processes, possibly associated with an inhibitory influence of emotional origin on the involuntary nervous system that, in part, mediates the outpouring of the growth hormone.

Illness

In my twenty-two-year longitudinal study of Philadelphia children I have accepted the general principle that the "usual childhood illnesses" (measles, mumps, chickenpox) do not affect the growth potential of the child. They may slow him down a bit, at the time of the illness, but the effects are not permanent. There is some reason to use age three years as a cut-off point: before the age of three years the registry of health damage may be more marked and rebound may be slower.

An Iowa study of ninety children, aged five to six years, recorded all absences from school due to "illness" (as reported by the mother). This was over a one-year period. The children were measured in fall and in spring. There was no influence, either in absolute (size) or in relative (proportion) dimensions and "illness" frequency. In other words these children were in spring just where they should have been, growthwise, had there been no "illnesses" at all. This holds true for all of early and middle childhood.

In the earlier years there is an interesting correlation, namely, that there is a higher incidence of illnesses in fast-growing children. This suggests a possibly greater vulnerability in the early maturers and fast growers for each sex.

The severity of the illness is, of course, a factor to be considered. The Oxford Child Health Survey studied the growth and maturation of children who were ill in a given year and compared them with healthy children during that same year. The ill children were divided into two groups, "mild" and "severe." No child in the "severe" group was ill more than six weeks. Figure 47 shows the results: height growth was significantly retarded, skeletal maturation was not; the frequency of bone "scars of arrested growth" was also significantly increased. Acheson

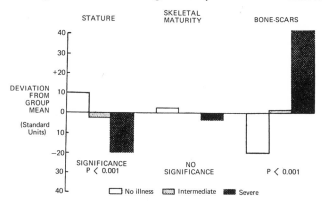

FIG. 47. Illness, Growth, and Maturation.

observes "that a very brief insult can greatly retard the growth of a child." Further, in this study, it was calculated that the "severe" height loss was the equivalent of an annual rate of ¼″, and there was no evidence of subsequent acceleration.

The Handicapped Child

The growth of handicapped children was recently studied by Pryor and Thelander. Four categories were set up: 1) Down's Syndrome ("Mongolism") which is due to a genetic (chromosomal) deviation; 2) multiple birth defects (congenital anomalies), coupled with various "environmental insults"; 3) cerebral palsy, with a history of birth trauma plus severe oxygen deprivation at birth (hypoxia); 4) neurologic handicaps, plus mild hypoxia at birth. These four groups are listed in their rank-order of severity. Group I was consistently below the average height for age and sex (for example, at age fifteen years the height-age was only eight or nine years), the head grew very little after three years of age, and infantile body proportions persisted; Group II was also below average height for age and sex, with the height curve lagging after age five; there was no adolescent spurt in growth; heads in both sexes were small for age; Group III grew pretty well until age ten and then slowed down noticeably, with no adolescent spurt. Group IV, which included children with "minimal brain damage," showed at all times a growth pattern well within normal range of variation.

Climate

There has been a spate of articles on the relation between growth and climate. In a study in Africa, a significant negative correlation was found between weight and average temperature. For children of both sexes the correlation coefficient is -0.706 at six years, -0.587 at ten years, and -0.525 at fourteen years; in adult males it is -0.600, in adult females, -0.809. The over-all body build of tropical dwellers of Africa (the Nilotic Negroes) is very linear with relatively long, slender arms and legs, especially in forearm and lower leg.

In 1942 Mills carried out experiments on the weight growth of mice, aged 3–21 weeks, under varying degrees of heat; control at $70°$–$75°$ F., cold room at $65°$F., and hot room at $90°$ F. The results are shown in Figure 48. The cold room mice grew as well as the control, but the hot room mice lagged far behind. Mills hypothesized that when the mice were in the hot room for a period of two weeks or longer, cellular combustion was reduced, possibly by some endocrine factor; the oxygen intake was

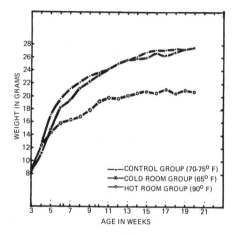

FIG. 48. Effect of Temperature upon Growth in Mice.

fifteen to twenty-five per cent less in these hot room mice. The endocrine hypothesis receives some support because the hot room mice were slowed ten per cent or more in the timing of their sexual cycles.

Mills then turned his attention to the growth of animals and humans in Panama. For example, he noted that it took four to five years to produce a nine-hundred-pound steer in tropical zone Panama and only one and a half to two years to grow a thousand-pound steer in temperate zone Iowa. He further reported that the need for thiamine for healthy growth (one of the vitamin B complexes) was twice as high at 90° than at 65°, on the basis of his experiments with mice. The slower rate of steer growth in the tropics was, he felt, a reflection of the greater thiamine need in a high temperature climate.

American-born white children in Panama, less than one year, were found to be taller than Panama-born white children. American children born in Panama were three per cent taller and ten per cent heavier than native Panamanian children (basically Indian plus Indian-white hybrids), but were two per cent shorter and three per cent lighter than children born in America and in Panama less than one year, Panama-born white American girls achieved the menarche somewhat later than white girls born in America.

The evidence brought forward in the foregoing paragraphs suggests that children born in the tropics grow and mature more slowly than those born in temperate zones. This is probably not a direct cause-and-effect relationship, for there is also to be considered a certain gross relationship between the more tropical climes and socioeconomic level, as well as of available foodstuffs. We cannot, in my opinion, take growth data from Africa and apply them willy-nilly to the growth of children in our own country. We do not have climatic extremes, but we do have a socio-economic dichotomy in industrial urban areas that contrasts "haves" with "have-nots."

Geography

The U.S. Public Health Service studied child growth in four geographic areas of the U.S.: 1) Northeast New England plus Middle Atlantic; 2) North Central Great Lakes; 3) South Central Lower Mississippi, from Kentucky to Texas; 4) Western (limited to Utah and Nevada). The children, age for age and by sex, were taller, area by area, from first to fourth, but there was no difference in incremental growth. These four areas, if one analyzes the ethnic or national make-up, merely reflect the genetically determined height of the ethnic strains involved. I see no reason to extol the salubrious "growth-promoting" value of the one area at the expense of deprecating the "growth-inhibiting" values of the other.

Race

The problem of racial growth in the United States focuses upon American white and American Negro children. Here, as far as it may be done, I shall consider the evidence for white and Negro children as representing two races. This is what the white child or the black child is born with, so to speak, as a representative of the Caucasoid and the Negroid groups of *Homo sapiens,* respectively.

All the anthropometric evidence at hand points to the fact that the Negro—both African and American—has a different body-build from the white—both European and American. The Negro has more of a linear build and is slender; the white has more of a lateral build and is stockier. This is a basic skeletal substructure, as may be seen in the construction of the pelvic girdle. The narrowed pelvis of the Negro has been likened to a "pedestal" for a narrow trunk; the broadened, flaring pelvis of the white has been likened to a "basin" for a broad torso. This is an important structural difference to note, for the more slender the build, the less weight per unit of height. Hence, if white weight and height standards are applied to Negro children the latter are apt to be penalized as being "underweight."

The data on the growth of African children reveal what seems to be a racially entrenched tendency to be born with a running start. Falkner and his associates studied the growth of West African children of Dakar from birth to two years of age. Males and females were heavier at birth and for the first six months than white newborns, then were lighter. Birth *length* in the Dakar children was a bit greater than in whites; *growth rate* was initially faster, but between six and nine months it began to slow, so that at one year the Dakar infants were shorter than whites. *Skeletal maturation* showed Dakar males and females to be developmentally equal at birth, but at six months female infants slowly forged ahead. When compared to white newborn the Dakar newborn were advanced, but here again a deceleration set in so that by one and a half years the Dakar infants were retarded in maturation age, for age and sex, as compared to whites.

Data on older Bantu children of South Africa, from seven to fifteen years of age, show that the slowed-up growth of the Negro child continues. The Bantu children in this age-bracket are shorter, lighter, with less subcutaneous fat as adduced from limb circumferences, and are, as expected, more linear or slender in over-all body-build. It has further been stated that African Negroes, in general, achieve adult stature later than in white adults: Negro males two years later, Negro females one and a half years later.

Now, let us turn to data on the American Negro. The best data on the newborn and infant are those of Kasius *et al.* (1957), on Philadelphia Negro and white children. In the following tabulation WM = white male, WF = white female, NM = Negro male, NF = Negro female:

Group	Birth	3 mos.	6 mos.	1 yr.
		Weight (lbs)		
WM	7.53	13.45	18.05	23.47
WF	7.26	12.42	16.72	21.68
NM	7.38	13.49	17.67	22.76
NF	7.15	12.43	16.46	21.42
		Length (cm)		
Group	Birth	3 mos.	6 mos.	1 yr.
WM	50.39	61.03	67.89	76.75
WF	49.61	59.88	66.26	74.83
NM	50.12	61.19	67.90	76.87
NF	49.40	59.98	66.14	75.60

In *weight* the Philadelphia Negro children are a bit lighter than whites except at three months. In *length* the Philadelphia white children are a bit longer at birth, but at three months the Negro children have caught up; at six months Negro and white children are about even, but by one year the Negro children, especially the females, are a bit longer. These are longitudinal data in that all children were measured for the first postnatal year.

Pooled data on the American Negro child generally substantiates the above interpretation. Birth *weight* in the American Negro child is four per cent less than that for whites, but at one year weight is only 2 per cent less.

Birth *length* in the American Negro child is two per cent less than that for whites, but from six months and on the length is about the same. Negro newborns tend to show a higher percentage of weights below 2,500 gms than whites (WM $= 6\%$, WF $= 6\%$, NM $= 8\%$, NF $= 16\%$).

The biological advancement of the Negro newborn child, as assessed via the criterion of skeletal or maturation age, is an interesting and provocative phenomenon. As I said earlier, this betokens a birth "head-start," which, however, is soon dissipated. The act of birth says, in effect, *go,* while the environment says *slow down.* Why there is this racial priority in the Negro newborn is not clear. I have pondered if this may be due to a natural selection, for the more rigorous total environment in which the African Negro child has for generations been born (a racial heritage in the American Negro newborn child, carried over from his African ancestry). If this hypothesis is true then the Hottentot Bushman newborn child of South Africa and the Australian aboriginal newborn child—both reared in a tough desert environment—should also be maturationally advanced.

IX

INHERITANCE FACTORS IN PHYSICAL GROWTH

The Ground Rules

I am sure we have all been present when a newborn baby is being viewed, proudly, by parents and relatives, especially grandparents. The babe is fondly appraised somewhat as follows: "He has his mother's lovely eyes," or "He has his daddy's mouth and chin," or ears or nose, or lips, and so on. And grandfather will see evidence of his family-line, or grandmother her family-line . . . and aunts and uncles will also see family resemblances. The baby boy or girl is seen as a wonderful combination of traits passed on by Dad (let's call him Mr. Smith) and Mother (Mrs. Smith, *née* Jones). Thus it is that the Smith family and the Jones family share in the creation of a new life.

This joyful summing-up of whom the babe resembles is a recognition of the fact that physical traits are inherited, that they have a genetic basis, and that they are passed on by the maternal family-line and paternal family-line. Let us look at this statement and analyze it for the general assumption it makes.

First, to pick out specific physical traits as eye color, nose shape, lip contour, chin shape, and so forth, is to regard them as discrete or *unit traits*. Each physiognomic characteristic is regarded as hereditarily transmissible, as though each were a single trait, each contributing its unique share to the ensemble of the baby-face. In principle this is true: each *does* contribute to the whole, each *is* part of a unique recombination of heritable Smith and Jones facial characteristics. A newborn babe is something brand-new, who will look like himself alone, and will resemble the parents and brothers and sisters, but will not be identical in appearance with them (the one exception is, of course, identical twins).

Second, to ascribe a given trait as a Smith or Jones resemblance, is to assume that that trait is *dominant,* i.e., that it has a positive strength, that it is genetically triumphant in its actual registry in the babe's face. Let us assume that Mother (a Jones) has blue eyes, and that Father (a Smith) has brown eyes. If the baby (at about six months of age) has Father's brown eyes it is because brown has dominated over blue. But what has happened to Mother's blue eyes? They are *recessive,* genetically submerged by the dominant brown eyes. They are figuratively in the background. The babe still carries them in his total genetic make-up, but they are hidden (actually, they are latent).

Third, there is an assumption that brown eyes or blue eyes are transmitted as genetically "pure," that Father has a genetic background for brown eyes only, Mother for blue eyes only. Actually, this is not true, for we've just noted that the brown-eyed baby has blue eyes somewhere in his hereditary background. It is more nearly correct that we think in terms of brown eyes seen, blue not seen or suppressed. I am aware that this is a vastly oversimplified way of looking at it, for eye color is a very complex phenomenon. Let us assume that two brown-eyed persons marry: let B = brown, b = blue (not brown); each person will be dominant for B, recessive for b; each will contribute B-ness and b-ness to the offspring; this gives two variables, taken twice, B and b from the male, B and b from the female.

$$Bb + Bb$$
$$BB$$
$$\left.\begin{matrix} Bb \\ Bb \end{matrix}\right\}$$
$$bb$$

Here two B's can get together to give one *BB;* BB and bb can get together to give two *Bb*'s; and two b's can get together to give one *bb*. As a result we have three brown-eyed (BB, 2 Bb) since B is dominant, and one blue-eyed (bb) since b is recessive. This is the 3:1 ratio made famous in Mendel's classic work with garden peas. The three brown-eyed and one blue-eyed are *what we see* —this is called the *phenotype.*

But there is a further step to take, for the three brown-eyed are alike only in appearance, but not in actual genetic make up. The three therefore are divided into one BB and two Bb; the BB has a "double dose" for brown, the two Bb's only a "single dose." It is possible to say, in effect, that BB is "pure," Bb is "mixed." In the same manner the bb may be said to be "pure." Now we have lost the 3:1 phenotypic ratio and have instead a 1:2:1 ratio ("pure" brown, "mixed" brown, "pure" blue, respectively). This is what is genetically present, the *genotype.* Another way of saying "pure" and "mixed" is to say BB is *homozygous* dominant, Bb, *heterozygous* dominant, and bb *homozygous* recessive.

From the foregoing discussion, it is obvious that BB × BB can give only BB, Bb × Bb must give BB, 2Bb, bb, and bb × bb can give only bb. In a real sense, "like begets like."

So much for the assumptions of unit traits, of dominance and recessive, and of inherent genetic make-up in terms of "pure" and "mixed." How do they apply to ourselves? Or, better, how much do we know about these things in human beings? The answers are pretty well qualified: there are no real single unit traits; simple dominance is rare (seen, for example, in achondroplastic dwarfism); simple recessiveness is also rare (seen, for example, in albinism); we know only a few genotypes (true genetic make-up) especially for the blood-group, and, a bit less clearly, for fingerprints.

By far the great bulk of genetic knowledge for man is based on the phenotype. We judge by what we see, rather than actually knowing, in terms of precise genetic make-up. In a way, ours is a surface-knowledge rather than an in-depth knowledge. For example, in a given child, here is an idea of what he or she receives from just *one side of the family:*

	% Contributed	Generation
Father	50%	2
Grandfather	25%	3
Great grandfather	12.5%	4
Great-great grandfather	6.12%	5
Great-great-great grandfather	3.06%	6
Great-great-great-great grandfather	1.53%	7
Great-great-great-great-great grandfather	0.77%	8

The chances are that not much will be attributable or recognizable beyond generation four (great grandfather). There is "thinning out" as the influence goes back in generational time.

Stature

As we study the growth of the child there are several principle themes: rate of dimensional growth and relation to parental size; age of achieving puberty and the "adolescent growth spurt"; the rate of maturational progress; and sex differences in amount (size) and rate (timing) of growth.

In general, large parents have large children. Birth size is related to the size of both parents, but there is a higher correlation of the fat-free weight of the child with the fat-free weight of the mother. From birth the parent-child resemblance increases to early midchildhood, at years five to seven. Then there may be a tapering-off in degree of similarity. Garn points out that "it is an important fact that infants relatively large during the first year may become relatively smaller as they grow toward adulthood."

The body length correlation or relationship between parent and child is a bit higher for father-son than for mother-son; it is considerably higher for mother-daughter than for father-daughter. In Figure 49 is shown the age-changes in height correlation for father-son, F/S, mother-daughter, M/D, father-daughter, F/D, and mother-son, M/S.

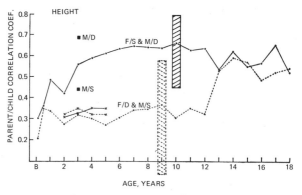

FIG. 49. Age-Changes in Parent-Child Correlation in Height.

Researchers at the Fels Institute for Child Growth in Yellow Springs, Ohio, have stressed the relation of the child to the midparent (father ht. + mother ht./2). The midparent-son correlation is higher at birth than for midparent-daughter; after that, especially in midadolescence, the midparent-daughter relationship is a bit greater. Selected birth to 18:0 year data for boys and girls as related to midparental statures are tabulated on page 157.

When siblings are compared for size the relationship is higher for sister-sister than for brother-brother, and both of these are higher than for brother-sister. The sister-sister size-growth relationship is highest between 5:0–

Midparental Height (cm)*

GIRLS

Age	161	163	165	167	169	171	173	175	177	178
B	47.3	48.9	49.0	49.2	49.2	48.8	49.7	49.1	49.0	47.5
5:0	106.8	103.5	108.9	109.9	109.1	111.6	110.9	111.0	112.6	111.7
10:0	136.0	135.1	139.0	140.3	136.9	143.8	142.9	143.1	143.8	143.6
15:0	155.9	159.8	162.6	163.7	162.2	164.0	167.1	168.4	165.0	166.5
18:0	156.2	161.0	165.0	167.2	164.3	164.4	167.9	171.8	165.7	170.8

BOYS

Age	161	163	165	167	169	171	173	175	177	178
B	—	47.1	49.7	50.3	50.0	48.3	50.7	50.0	51.5	51.4
5:0	—	105.6	108.5	110.6	110.0	111.5	113.2	112.7	114.6	113.8
10:0	—	132.5	135.8	138.8	137.4	139.8	143.8	141.5	145.3	143.2
15:0	—	165.8	168.1	169.1	167.9	172.9	173.0	174.7	176.4	175.2
18:0	—	171.5	175.0	177.9	176.2	180.5	180.2	178.6	177.6	186.3

*2.54 cm = one inch

10:0 years, while that of brother-brother peaks at 12:0 years, then rapidly decreases.

It is safe to make the following generalization for stature: mother-child correlation tends to be higher than father-child; in both parent-child sets the correlation is higher in early adolescence; there is little or no correlation between parental height and the *timing* of the "growth spurt," though there is a slight correlation between parental height and *amount* of height growth of the child in early adolescence. My former teacher, T. Wingate Todd, used to say that at nine or ten years adult proportions are forecast: the boy is father to the man, the girl mother to the woman.

Body-Build and Maturation

The best data on body dimensions are from the Ohio (Fels Institute) research group. Transverse chest dimensions (on the bony rib-cage) were measured on postero-anterior chest X-ray films. A dimension above the mean was scored as L (large) and one below the mean as S (small). There were twenty LL and fifteen SS parents, with fifty-six and thirty-one children, respectively. The bony chest measurement is a good one for it is significantly correlated with the fat-free "lean body mass" and is only slightly correlated with stature. Some very interesting facts have emerged:

1. The LL *boys* surpassed the SS boys in both height and weight growth from birth to 17:0 years; the height relationship in LL boys was highest at 5:5–13:0 years, the weight at 1:0–17:0 years.
2. The LL *girls* showed the same tendency as did the LL boys, though the absolute LL-SS differences were smaller in girls. The height relationship in LL girls was highest at 5:0–7:0 years, only, while the weight relationship was highest at 5:0–9:0 years and again at 17:0 years.
3. The LL children were maturationally advanced over the SS children at 1:6, 3:0, and 11:0 years, as deter-

mined by assessment of ossification seen in X-ray films of the hand.

4. In motor behavior the LL children were advanced over the SS children in scores on the Gesell test at 0:6 months, 1:0 year, and 1:6 years; in the Merrill-Palmer tests they scored higher at 1:6 and 2:0, as well as in the early Stanford-Binet quotients.

5. Genes for body-build also influence *rate* of maturation, i.e., LL children are more often "early maturers."

Within body-build there is evidence that certain components are also inherited: there are, for example, lightly and heavily muscled lineages (a case in point is the reduced calf circumference of the Negro, both in childhood and in adulthood). Children who are maturationally advanced in the first year of life lose fat earlier than in delayed children; gain in muscle mass is apparently genetic, for identical twins are significantly more alike in this respect than fraternal twins or siblings.

There is no doubt that "early," "average" and "late" maturers run in families. This in turn relates to timing of height growth. In Figure 50 the height-growth curves of three sisters are shown, to the left plotted against

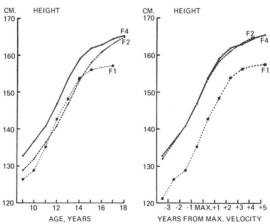

FIG. 50. Height-Growth Curves in Three Sisters (see text for details).

chronological age, to the right against time of maximum height velocity (MHV). When this is done the curves for sisters F_2 and F_4 are coincident.

We may conclude that while bone size has a genetic basis, actual bone growth is dependent upon adequate nutrition.

The Teeth

The teeth are beyond a doubt under a definite amount of genetic control. In 1967 I reviewed the literature on the subject especially with reference to family-line inheritance, and racial data. There are two major aspects of dental development to consider, namely, calcification of the tooth in its bony socket, and eruption of the tooth into the dental arch for functional use. The two processes are, of course, related, for as the tooth calcifies (cusps, crown, neck, root) it slowly emerges from its socket to take its place as a "cutter" or "grinder" in the upper and lower arches.

Again, we employ the by now familiar analysis of correlations or relationships within the family; parents with children, children with brothers and sisters. There is a high sibling correlation for crown calcification, root growth, and eruption movement of the tooth as it "cuts the gum" and aligns itself in the tooth row in each arch; the relationship is higher for sister-sister than for brother-brother. It is worthy of note that for all aspects of dental development the correlation is higher intra-girl than intra-boy. All this suggests that the sex difference is a real one, influenced by the extra X chromosome of the female. And this may possibly explain the more frequent crowding or rotation of teeth in girls than in boys, which, in turn, predisposes to malocclusion.

Size of teeth, sequence and time of calcification and eruption, certainly run in families, in varying degrees of genetic control.

As far as race differences are concerned it can be stated that Europeans and American whites are later in time of eruption than some Asiatics, American Indians, Eskimos, and the American Negro; an extreme is reached in that in some African tribes the third permanent molar (which we call the "wisdom tooth" and which in us erupts at 18:0–20:0 years +) may erupt at 12:0–13:0 years.

The problem of *missing teeth* is a fascinating one. In about two hundred million years the mammals (the zoological class to which we belong) have gone from sixty-six teeth to forty-four at one hundred million years ago, and to thirty-two at sixty million years ago. We have thirty-two permanent teeth, eight incisors, four canines, eight premolars, and twelve molars; the incisors are front teeth, the canines are corner teeth, and the premolars-molars, front to back, are cheek teeth. In about ten million years (or a few million more) we'll be reduced to twenty teeth (assuming man survives that long). Certain of our teeth are on the way out, for they are often congenitally missing, i.e., they never did start to form in the fetus. Here's a schema of what's happening (I = incisor, C = canine, P = premolar, M = molar, S = stable, V = variable, $+$, $++$ and $++(+)$ = degree of variability); the left side of the tooth rows only is shown, upper and lower, permanent or second set:

S	V+	S	S	V	S	V	V++
I_1	I_2	C	P_1	P_2	M_1	M_2	M_3
I_1	I_2	C	P_1	P_2	M_1	M_2	M_3
V	S	S	S	V	S	V	V++(+)

The third molars are the most variable, the lower a bit more than the upper; next comes the upper I_2; then, not in an absolute order, lower I_1, upper and lower P_2, and upper and lower M_2. We are losing one incisor, one premolar, and two molars—instead of a dental formula of 2I–1C–2P–3M we will have 1I–1C–1P–1M.

When one to four third molars are missing it is part of a polymorphism, i.e., its absence has a genetic growth effect on the other teeth; a person with one to four M_3's missing has other teeth absent thirteen times more often than where all four M_3's erupt; furthermore, the other teeth are delayed in calcification and eruptive movement.

The missing upper I_2 (missing most frequently after the M_3), presents a fascinating problem. Often it is not entirely missing, but is represented by a small, conical "peg" or just a rudimentary nubbin. This tooth may have a very important "marker" role; lateral to it is the C, and between the upper I_2 and upper C there is a bone-suture, i.e., the line of demarcation between the premaxillary bone (bearing I_1–I_2) and the maxillary bone (bearing C, P_1–$_2$, M_1–$_3$). This suture line is often the site of a cleft, involving the alveolar bone (the part where the teeth are socketed). Therefore, there are some geneticists who feel that a missing upper I_2 is a sign of a tendency to palatal clefting. In other words, often when only the missing upper I_2 is involved, the person "just missed" having a cleft. This is spoken of as a tendency to clefting of a low degree of expressivity.

Cleft Palate and Cleft Lip

Sometime between the forty-ninth and fifty-fifth day after conception the tongue of the embryo drops from between the right and left palatal shelves, laterally placed, and these begin to move to the mid-line to form a complete bar of bone between the oral and nasal cavities; this bar of bone is the *hard palate*. Behind it are muscles and connective tissue that make up the *soft palate,* which functions in swallowing and in speech. In about 1 in 800 times something goes wrong: the palate is incomplete and is said to be "cleft." From behind forward, in the midline, first the uvula, then the soft palate, then the hard palate may be cleft; this is about two thirds of the way forward; then either right or left, or both, premaxillary-maxillary sutures may be open (cleft) involving the alveolar or socket bone between the upper lateral incisor (milk or i2, later permanent or I2) and canine (milk or c, later permanent or C). The lip may also be cleft, either right or left, or both. Lip may be cleft alone or in association with cleft palate. Cleft lip and cleft palate do not necessarily go together, although cleft lip and cleft alveolar are more frequently associated than cleft lip and cleft soft palate or cleft of posterior two-thirds hard palate.

The question arises: is clefting of palate and/or lip hereditary? The answer is not clear. In the experimental animal (rat, mouse, monkey) a "teratogen" at a critical embryonic moment may cause cleft. Teratogens are found in certain nutritional deficiencies, or in endocrine and chemical imbalances, or in physical circumstances, as local anoxia (not enough oxygen) or in radiation of the female carrying the young. In humans one of the most dire causes is rubella, or German measles, whose toxin is a potent teratogen.

Thus, anything untoward—anoxia (which may be caused by maternal anesthetization), radiation, nutritional inadequacy, illness (rubella, especially)—in the first three months of pregnancy (the first trimester) should at once be reported to the obstetrician.

Now let us look at some English family histories on clefting reported by Drillien and associates in 1966. In twenty families of patients with cleft palate only, twenty-five relatives had a cleft lip and/or cleft palate: sixty-eight per cent of the affected relatives had cleft palate only; twenty-four per cent had cleft lip with or without cleft palate; on eight per cent there were no data. In thirty families of patients with cleft lip (with or without cleft palate) forty-eight relatives were similarly affected; eighty-one per cent of the affected relatives had cleft lip (with or without cleft palate); seventeen per cent had cleft palate only; on two per cent there were no data. In general, half of the relatives of patients with cleft lip + cleft palate were similarly affected; a quarter had cleft lip only; a quarter had cleft palate only.

One more word is to be here added, namely that often cleft palate is part of a complex (a syndrome) of congenital defects. This is called a "genetic pleiotropism." Because of this fact, whenever a case history of cleft palate (with or without cleft lip) is being worked up, it is necessary to probe the family history in depth for *other* —and possibly associated—birth defects.

The most conservative conclusion is that cleft palate and/or lip *does* seem to run in families. If, for example, a grandparent or great uncle or aunt, or a cousin—indeed, any member of the extended family (the paternal and maternal family-lines)—has had a cleft lip and/or palate then the chance of recurrence is greater than if the family history were one hundred per cent negative. However, lip or palate, or both, may be cleft with no family history, either via a genetic mutation or a teratogen.

The Chromosome

A "chromosome" is literally a "color body" for it takes a specific stain. More precisely it is any of several thread-like bodies, made up of chromatin, and found in a cell nucleus; the chromosome carries the genes in a linear order. Man has forty-six chromosomes. Two of these are sex chromosomes: XX for female, XY for male.* The other forty-four chromosomes are called autosomes and carry genes other than for sex.

If male and female are crossed (mated) the result is as follows:

*The X and the Y are simply identifying letters. The X was named first, much as was the X in X-ray. Then when it was seen with another chromosome (not an X) the other was called Y.

Male \ Female	X	X
X	XX	XX
Y	XY	XY

The result is two XX, two XY, a 1:1 ratio of two females, two males.

In recent years it has been possible, via tissue culture, to study the chromosomal pattern of an individual via a process called "karyotyping" (see Figure 51). As a result

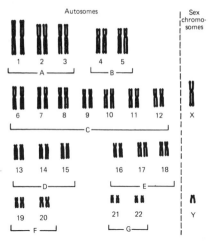

FIG. 51. Human Chromosomes (Arranged According to the Denver Convention).

we now know much more about genetic mechanisms. There are many kinds of chromosomal aberrations. We shall here note only a few of the more frequent:

Klinefelter's Syndrome, XXY (an extra X)
The patient has a male phenotype, with gynecomastia (breast development), sparse facial hair, a high-pitched voice, and small testes.

Turner's Syndrome, XO (one X missing)
   The patient has a female phenotype, with short stature,
   primary amenorrhea (no menstruation) and very weak
   or absent secondary sex traits.

   In recent months much has been made of the XYY
individual, a male; it is believed that the XYY male is
plus-prone to violent criminal behavior, especially since
significantly more XYY males are in maximum security
prisons (or hospitals) than would be expected from
chance alone. However, less than five per cent of all
living XYY's have been confined as above. One is inclined
to rate the environmental stimulus and/or opportunity to
criminal violence equally high.
   The best known of the chromosomal aberrations is that
in the Downs Syndrome (popularly called "mongolism").
These individuals have 47 chromosomes; two sex chromosomes XX or XY, and forty-five autosomes. The extra
autosome is "Trisomy 21," i.e., chromosome #21 is triple
instead of the normal double. The chromosomal aberrations are due to faulty cell division when male and female
sex cells get together.
   The over-all chance of an American female having a
Downs child is 1:680. At age twenty years it is 1:700, but
by age 40–45 the chances are greatly increased, varyingly
stated as 1:50 to 1:20. It is not certain if parity (age-order
of the child) is a factor, but maternal age surely is.
   The Downs child presents a characteristic picture, so
much so that it has been said that all Downs children
look more alike than any one of them looks like his own
parents. They are short-statured, and become progressively more so from birth to 15:0 years; this shortness is
primarily in the legs, so that the trunk/limb ratio remains
more infantile. The head is small, for it almost ceases to
grow by about age three years; head length growth is inhibited more than breadth growth; as a result the Downs
youngster is quite round-headed. The ear is small, especially in length, in some cases it is vestigial. Facial growth
lags in height and breadth; it, too, remains infantile. Nose

root is depressed and the nose often looks like a "baby nose." In the inner corner of the eye there is a vertical eye fold known as the median epicanthic fold. It is this trait which makes for a slant-eye—hence, the term "mongol" or "mongoloid." Trunk dimensions are close to normal for sex and age. The body build is stocky. In all dimensions males are more variable than females; that is why the Downs girls are more "look-alikes" than the Downs boys.

Downs children are mentally retarded in varying degree. Most are educable, mainly in a vocational direction involving a certain amount of manual dexterity. They have a good memory for detail in various experienced situations and for music. Most are cheerful, very friendly, and very good in imitative behavior and/or mimicry.

Twins

Identical twins (monozygotic or one-egg) are always like-sexed (two boys or two girls), fraternals (dizygotic or two-egg) may be like-sexed or brother-sister (see Figure 52). I write about twins with keen interest, for I have a fraternal twin brother. We represent what so frequently happens with fraternals: there is a sibling resemblance, but essentially I follow the paternal line, he the maternal.

There is no doubt that twinning is hereditary, dizygotic perhaps a bit more so than monozygotic, i.e., they run in families, and in *both* sides of the family. The chances of producing twins is greater in brothers of twinning fathers and sisters of twinning mothers. Twins share in the general rule that mortality is higher in plural births, and that prematurity is relatively frequent. Often, at birth, one twin is larger than the other.

In 1967 the U.S. Public Health Service published data on twins (Publ. #1,000, Series 21, No. 14). Of 27.9 million live births in the U.S., 1960–1966, only 557,000 (2%) were from plural births where one child was born alive. All but 7,800 of these were twins. In 1960–1966 one of

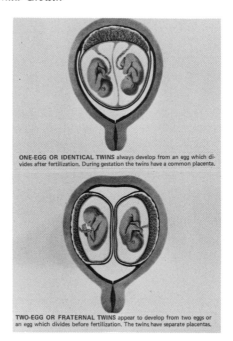

ONE-EGG OR IDENTICAL TWINS always develop from an egg which divides after fertilization. During gestation the twins have a common placenta.

TWO-EGG OR FRATERNAL TWINS appear to develop from two eggs or an egg which divides before fertilization. The twins have separate placentas.

FIG. 52. Scheme of One-Egg (Identical) and Two-Egg (Fraternal) Twins.

every 51 babies born alive was a twin, and one of every 3,600 was a triplet, a "quad" or a "quint." Since twins result from a single multiple delivery the probability of twins is one in 100.

This sets the stage for the "Hellin-Zeleny Hypothesis": if a pair of twins occurs once in 100 deliveries then triplets $= n^2$, quadruplets $= n^3$, and quintuplets $= n^4$. If we accept 1 in 100 as twins, then 1 in 100^2 (10,000) = triplets, 1 in 100^3 (1,000,000) = quadruplets, and 1 in 100^4 (100,000,000) = quintuplets; this is the "rule of n" (100).

Multiple births are more frequent in nonwhites (25.8 per 1,000 live births) than in whites (18.8 per 1,000 live births). They are least frequent in mothers under 20 years, rise to a peak at 35–39 years, and decrease after 40 years. In whites plural births are 11.6 per 1,000 live births among teen-age mothers, 27.8 per 1,000 live births in mothers of 35–39 years, at 13.5 per 1,000 live births in mothers 45+ years. All along, plural births are more frequent in nonwhites.

Ever since the days of Castor and Pollux, Romulus and Remus, there has been built up a folklore on twins; they even figure in astronomy and astrology. Here are a few facts and figures:

1. The best method of establishing that twins are identical is by fingerprints: the prints of at least seven fingers will have identical patterns.
2. Like-sexed twins occur twice as often as unlike-sexed.
3. Twins are not more apt to have twins than are nontwins.
4. Left-handedness is more frequent in twins (particularly identicals): fifteen per cent are left-handed as compared to seven per cent in the total population.
5. The likelihood of twins increases with birth-order: after two children the odds increase by thirty per cent; after five children they increase by two hundred per cent.
6. Most twins are born to mothers aged 30:0–34:0 years.
7. Older men are more apt to father twins: mothers aged 30:0–34:0 years have twice the chance of having twins if the father is over 35:0 years of age.
8. Twins are not necessarily conceived at the same time: fraternal twins may be born a week or two apart; they may even have different fathers (a case in point: one twin was white, the other Negro).
9. Twins often are late in starting to talk. They relate to one another so closely that often they develop their own "language," partly sign, partly unique vocalizations.
10. Twins are two *individuals*. There is a temptation "to be fair" and to "treat them exactly alike." This may

often submerge the individuality of each. Fraternals are apt to show greater sibling rivalry than identicals, but in all instances twins are one + one, *each* entitled to his own full measure of individual self-expression in all things—in behavior patterns, likes and dislikes, clothing, and so on.

Facial Features

Quite apart from similarities in twins is the major question of heredity in various measured traits in all children, particularly physiogomic traits, i.e., the complex of physical traits of head and face: hair, eye, ears, nose, mouth and lips, chin, cheeks, and so on (see Scheinfeld, 1965).

In the *hair* dark color is dominant over light and red is recessive to all others. White hair (so-called "platinum blonde," apart from the depigmented hair of later years) has two "white" genes, recessive to all others; it may or may not be associated with albinism. Blonde hair has two "yellow" genes, with additional diluted melanin (dark pigment). The genetics of red hair is not clear. Brown hair has two "brown" genes or one brown + one yellow or one brown + one red. Black hair is a matter of the intensity of two pairs of dark brown genes, or brown genes + the genes of any lighter shade. Hair form is probably polygenic, i.e., many genes. In general, straight hair is dominant in a cross. If St = straight, Cu = curly, Wa = wavy we may have in white children the following: St × St = St; St × Cu = St + Cu, St × Wa = St + Wa, Cu × Wa = St + Wa + Cu. So-called woolly or kinky hair is dominant over all others. The occipital hair-whorl (on the back of the head) probably has a single pair of genes. A clockwise whorl is recessive to counter-clock: seventy per cent have counter-clock, twenty-five per cent have clockwise, five per cent have both (a real problem in hair-combing!). It has been said that the gene locus for the occipital hair whorl is on the same chromosome as that for missing third permanent molars.

In the *eyes,* also, dark color is dominant over light, but the pigmentation problem involves many complex considerations of the intricacy of the structure of the eyes; so complicated is this that the genotypes for eye color are only conjectural. Blue eyes are really an optical illusion of light reflected from pigment granules back of the iris. There are said to be two "blue" genes; one alone is recessive to all others save those for albinism. Genes for green and gray eyes are unknown. Brown-black eyes have two "brown" genes or one brown + one of a lighter shade. Albino eyes are recessive to all others; they are due to double genes for albinism. For the soft parts of the eyes it may be said that a straight eye-slit (palpebral fissure) is dominant over an oblique; a medial eye-fold (inner corner) is dominant over a fold of the eyelid.

Turning now to soft parts of head and face it may be noted that in the *ear* a free ear-lobe is dominant over an attached lobe, and that a simple or slight helical fold (the fold of the free hinder part of the ear) is dominant over a complex or extensive fold (the simple fold is negroid, the complex fold, white). In the *nose* a prominent, convex nose is dominant over a straight nose or a concave nose (a "ski nose" or "tip-tilted nose"); a high narrow bridge is dominant over a broad low bridge (a high-bridged aquiline nose is white, a low-bridged broad nose with flared nostrils is negroid). In the *mouth* and *chin* area it may be observed that chin height, and upper and lower lip heights (both integumental and mucous or vermilion) are due to many genes with no dominance. A thick, everted lower lip ("Hapsburg lip") is dominant. A "cleft chin"—vertical depression in the midline—and a "grooved chin"—horizontal depression below the lower lip—are simple dominants. Total mouth breadth, per se, and mouth breadth as a ratio of lip height, show no recognizable genetic mediation. In general thin, slight to moderately everted lips are white, while thick, moderately to markedly everted lips are negroid. The latter complex seems to dominate in a cross, but as a whole, lip thickness is almost as variable intra-racially as it is inter-racially. A *dimple* in the cheek is dominant.

Radiation

A discussion of genetics and growth would be incomplete without mention of radiation. I shall not even try to discuss the problem, for it is emotional and fear-packed for one thing, and for another we have only one fact to conjure with, namely that in the experimental animal radiation *can* cause genetic damage (mutations).

In 1957 the World Health Organization concluded of radiation that "a threshold dose does not exist for genetic change." Dosage is measured in roentgen units, referred to as *r;* obviously, too many *r*'s are a genetic threat: frequency of congenital abnormalities; frequency of miscarriages and stillbirths; variations in the sex ratio. The use of the X-ray machine poses a threat, especially if the gonadal areas are involved (ovaries in the female, testes in the male). It is recommended by W.H.O. that gonadal dosage in an individual be limited to five *r*'s per year, and that total dosage from conception to 30:0 years of age is not to exceed 50 *r*'s (the International Committee on Radiological Protection would cut this to 10*r*).

In our time the major radiation threat is that from nuclear explosion fall-out. In 1953 teams of the Atomic Energy Commission of the U.S. issued reports on preliminary findings on survivors at Hiroshima or Nagasaki. Data gathered in 1950 on children who survived the blast still showed "adverse" growth effects: they were retarded in height, weight, and skeletal maturation; boys more so than girls. It was pointed out, however, that this retardation may have had multiple causes: thermal or other radiation; physical injuries; the psychological trauma of the bomb-drop; the severe socio-economic disruption following the blast. Studies of children born to survivors of the atomic bombing of Hiroshima and Nagasaki showed no increase in birth defects, and a slight increase in the number of stillbirths. Birth weight of children born to exposed parents was not definitely affected. The general feeling was that in this first post-Bomb generation it was doubtful if the genetic effects of the radiation would show up "in full strength."

Heredity vs. Environment

There is a time-honored cliché, heredity vs. environment, which may appear guised as "endogenous vs. exogenous," or "inherent vs. acquired," or any similar comparison that pits genetic causation against environmental modification. As one goes through the literature on human genetics, particularly the references on the phenotype, one comes to the feeling that oft is it impossible to say, "here genetics ends, environment begins." Look at this example (by McKusick, from Hammons, 1959) concerning hardening of the arteries:

Multifactorial Causation of Atherosclerosis

At the top of this chart are possible genetic factors, at the bottom factors of environmental impact.

The horizontal dotted line, right and left, is a presumed heredity-environment boundary. Here the end-result is atherosclerosis, the result of the warp of heredity *plus* (not vs.) the woof of environment.

Child growth is human growth, and that means that it is characteristic of man—the most adaptable creature on earth; more than that, he has adapted so much, both for good and for bad, to himself. That is why human child growth should be so carefully cared for and nurtured, both pre- and postnatally. The environment, in the early developmental periods, can cut so deeply that it may cause severe and lasting—even irreversible—effects: it may facilitate, but it may also mar. The environment of the growing child must give free opportunity to maximum variability, for "diversity is an essential aspect of functionalism."

X

THE MOTOR USE OF THE BODY:
POSTURE, EXERCISE, SPORTS

Basic Motor Patterns

The month-old embryo has a definite trunk from which, at appropriate levels, two pairs of lobelike "limbs" have projected laterally. These are the future arms and legs, with hand, forearm, upper arm, and foot, lower leg, thigh, respectively. In infancy the creeping or crawling child is basically a quadruped, even though he later is an upright biped: right foot and left hand are on the ground together, then the left foot and right hand. This pattern will persist. Check yourself while walking: as the right foot comes down the left arm swings out, and as the left foot descends the right arm is forward in position.

There is another way in which the newborn baby is a quadruped, namely in the vertebral column or backbone. At first the backbone is arched in a single large curve. In a quadruped, a horse for example, the backbone is arched upward; the spines of the anterior vertebrae are slanted towards the rump, while those of the posterior vertebrae are slanted towards the head and neck; as a result at mid-back level there is a meeting of backward directed—forward directed forces while walking. In front are the forelegs, in back the hindlegs, each as sort of foundations for what William King Gregory has called "the bridge that walks"—the total quadrupedal skeleton is constructed like a cantilever bridge.

In the newborn baby, when he is on his belly, the back-bone does in fact arch upward (however, the direction of the vertebral spines all tend to be backward, which is an adaptation to locomotion on the hind legs). With growth, by the end of the first year or so, the backbone loses its single arched curve, and the distinctly human "S-curve" manifests itself: in the cervical or neck region the curve is convex forward (called a lordosis); in the thoracic or shoulder-chest region the curve is convex backward (called a kyphosis); in the lumbar region ("the small of the back") the curve is convex forward (lordosis); finally, in the sacral region at buttock level, the curve is convex backward (kyphosis). From above down, neck to rump, there is lordosis-kyphosis-lordosis-kyphosis. This is the evolved bipedal mechanism, adapted to arms for manipulation and legs for walking. The backbone is now characteristically human, ready for all the stress- and weight-bearing forces that will arise in human activities and locomotion. Our arms and legs and our backbones are the human heritage of millions of years of evolution; in a sense in prenatal life and in the first year of postnatal life, we recapitulate the evolutionary step (a small step for the baby, but a giant step for evolution).

As the baby creeps, crawls, cruises, pulls itself up, and finally walks, the mother has facilitated the developmental progress. Studies have shown that learning progress in the child, with reference not only to walking, but to all motor activities, is faster in a first-born baby and earlier where the mother is young. Obviously, the factor here is amount and kind of encouragement given the child, related to the available time of the mother. Other studies have shown that home-reared and institutionalized children develop motor skills at about the same rate up to five years of age; after that the home-reared children forge ahead, doing much better in the fine-muscle skills, especially.

Body Posture

A very illuminating study of flat feet is that of Morley who classified the arch of the foot via footprints (Figure 53). On the print a line (A) was drawn along the big-toe side of the foot; a line (B) perpendicular to (A) was

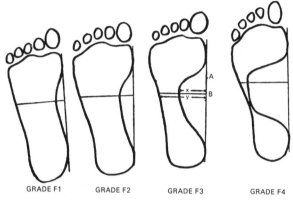

GRADE F1   GRADE F2   GRADE F3   GRADE F4

FIG. 53. Method of Grading Footprints for the Evaluation of Flat Feet.

drawn through the highest point of the arch as seen in the footprint; this will give a ratio of arch height (x) to foot width (y) $(\frac{x}{y})$. The scoring is as follows:

F1 = x is less than ¼ of y (flat foot)
F2 = x is ¼ to ½ of y (moderately flat)
F3 = x is ½–¾ of y (good arch)
F4 = x is ¾+ of y (high arch).

All babies have F1 = flat feet. This is entirely normal for the sole of the newborn has a fat pad that obscures the bony (tarso-metatarsal) arch. In a few years the fat pad will go and arch form assert itself. Some children will retain an infantile-like flatness (more often in Negro children), but most will move on to F4: F1 is seen to 3–4 years in twenty-five per cent of children, F2 at 4–6 years in sixty-five per cent, F3 at 6–9 years in eighty per cent, and F4 after that in about ninety to ninety-five per cent. This suggests that five to ten per cent of children will have flat feet to a greater or lesser degree on into the pre-pubertal period.

The problem of knock-knees has been studied not only by Morley, but by Robinow and his associates on the Fels Institute children. Two different methods of appraisal are employed, the one visual via standard photographs (Robinow), the other mensurational (Morley).

In Figure 54 are shown the photographs of children rated 1–6, from no knock-knees to marked.

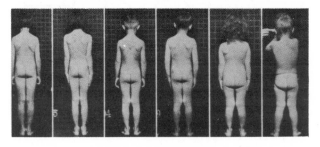

FIG. 54. Method of Grading Knock-Knees.

With the child lying down or sitting, and with lower leg at right angles to thigh, knees touching, the distance between the two medial malleoli (ankle bone on each big-toe side) was measured, and four grades set up: 1) inter-malleolar distance of less than 1″ (2.5 cm); 2) between 1″ and 2″ (5.0 cm); 3) 2″–3″ (7.5 cm); 4) 3″+. The frequency of knock-knees increases to 3–3¼ years at which time twenty-two per cent of children have a measurement of 2″ or more, which is grade 3); only twenty-six per cent had less than 1″ while fifty-two per cent had 1–2″. There were no sex differences under five years of age. In school children the incidence of knock-knees of 3″+ was the same for boys and girls, but "lesser amounts of knock-knees were more common amongst the girls." Knock-kneed children usually weigh more than like-sexed and like-aged children without knock-knees.

There is no evidence that knock-knees are related to flat feet, age of first walking, length of breast-feeding, vitamin supplementation in the first eighteen months, or illness (time spent in bed).

There are other postural variables that may be mentioned: hyperextended knees (legs "bent backward"); lumbar lordosis (marked forward curvature at the small-of-the-back area) so that the child looks "sway-backed" and "pot-bellied," "slumped back" or "round shouldered"; pronation, i.e., in standing the weight is born on the big-toe side of the foot and the heel is turned outwards. This gives the appearance of flat feet and conduces to knock-knees. All this is resolved by six to seven years of age. All of these are related to age (Figure 55): moderate lumbar

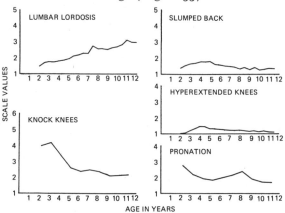

FIG. 55. Age-Changes in Various Postural Variables.

lordosis normally increases; "slumped back" is moderate at age two, then decreases; hyperextended knees are moderate at four years, then decrease; and pronation "peaks" at 3:0, and 8:0–9:0, and is moderate after that.

The judgment of "poor posture" is thus rather complex, for several postural variables are being evaluated, which are all, to a greater or less degree, interrelated. The over-all picture suggests strongly that inadequate muscle function is basic to the majority of postural variations and defects observed in children. This suggests that the growing child should be provided with every opportunity to use his entire body and so to develop gross and fine muscle skills and coordination. Age-related toys such as velocipedes, conveyances moved by pedaling (toy autos, etc.), and "jungle-gyms" with bars and rings, should be made available and their use encouraged. The preschool and school child who is a TV addict is more liable to postural problems than is the youngster outdoors playing "tag" or "catch" on a vacant lot or playground.

I would be in error were I to leave the impression that muscle function is the only answer to poor posture. Bowlegs, which have not been referred to, are more apt to be caused by malnutrition which in its severest form may cause rickets (rachitic bowing). In these days, with good nutrition and vitamin-D supplementation, rickets is almost unknown in the great group of middle-class people. Rickets is still found, of course, in the "misery spots" of the world. There is some evidence that flat feet run in families, but the data are not conclusive. On the whole, poor posture, however defined or localized, is most often environmental, related to bad habits of sitting, of relaxation, and of a slovenly regime of gross muscle use in all activities. Over and beyond this I add that if the poor posture, especially with reference to back and legs, persists after, say, seven years or so, an orthopedic physician should be consulted.

Exercise

Now we turn to the question of exercise and the growing child. In the United States there is no greater champion of physical fitness than Dr. Thomas Cureton, Professor of Physical Education at the University of Illinois and Coach-Advisor to the U.S. Olympic teams. Physical fitness and good health go hand-in-hand; a child (or adult) who so qualifies will the better stand stress; will resist fatigue; will resist the milder infections that may move in when fatigue is present; will have greater zest for life and a more balanced body-mind relationship. "Love of life" goes along with the vigorous play of the child and the satisfying occupation of time and energy in the adult.

How does exercise affect the growth of the child? The answer is that the growth-pattern may be facilitated in that full growth potential will be achieved. It does not *promote* growth in the sense that the child will be bigger, i.e., taller; nor will it *retard* growth in the sense that he will be "stunted," i.e., shorter. Exercise works more upon the compartments or components of the body than it does upon total linear growth. There is no doubt that exercise stimulates *muscle-development.*

Exercise studies with dogs give evidence that there is a hypertrophy (size increase) of individual muscle fibers, as opposed to the appearance of new fibers. The story is, in essence, not *more* muscle, but *increase in muscle mass* and in functional strength. Further, in the experimental set-ups, the greater the intensity and the longer the duration, the more the hypertrophy and the greater the contractile force of the muscle(s). Not more muscle, but *better* muscle!

It is impossible to study a single muscle in a child, but it is possible to measure the body before or after a regime of exercise, or to compare exercised vs. nonexercised groups. Simon (cited in Malina, 1969a) did a variation of the latter situation. Two groups of 14–15 year old children were studied: Group I received daily physical training; Group II received physical training twice a week. The period involved was six months.

Trait	Gains at end of experiment	
	I. *Daily Group*	II. *2/wk. Group*
Body length	1.10 cm	1.19 cm
Body weight	5.8 kg	7.8 kg
Shoulder width	2.4 cm	1.4 cm
Chest circumference	3.01 cm	0.98 cm
Diff. upper arm circ., elbow flexed and extended	1.5 cm	0.8 cm
Thigh circumference	2.3 cm	1.5 cm
Respiratory amplitude	5.5 cm	3.7 cm

The gains here are certainly in mass of the body parts measured, but not in body length, and the gains favor the more intensively trained children of Group I. In this same study there were similar differential gains in sports activities, as running, jumping, and throwing performances.

There are other studies of like nature, and emerging from them is what I consider the real and beneficial change, observable when body composition is measured: there is a significant increase in active (lean) tissue, with a corresponding reduction in fat tissue. This is tantamount to saying that exercise stimulates "healthier" (because more actively functional) tissue, rather than the far more inert fat tissues. There is reason to conclude that an exercise program, conscientiously followed, stimulates "growth" in the body parts or regions specifically exercised. I have put growth in quotes because I want it clearly understood that I do not mean height growth; I refer to the increased functional efficiency which results, and I hold this to be facilitative in the total growth process.

Studies of dominant vs. nondominant forearms in tennis, for example, have shown significantly greater muscle and bone changes in the dominant forearm. These players had begun practicing and playing in the 'teens and some writers have suggested that the bone "growth apparatus" was modified. If by this certain cellular and trabecular changes are meant, I tend to agree. But the "growth apparatus" in terms of linear growth or in rate of maturation, remains uninfluenced; these are too deeply rooted in constitutional and genetic make-up.

Now, I want to follow-up this business of exercise and bone. The facts of use hypertrophy and disuse atrophy are well established: in use the bone is larger, more rugged, better mineralized, with a thicker cortex, and so on; in disuse the bone may be shorter, less rugged (gracile or slender), demineralized, with a thinner cortex. In a sense there is an apparent contradiction here, in that bones are longer in use, shorter in disuse: the answer is that the use-bone is not longer than it would have been, but that the disuse-bone is shorter than it should have been. In other words use has facilitated growth potential, disuse stultified it.

I have studied skeletons with a unilateral arm or leg amputation, high up enough, in upper arm (humerus) or in thigh (femur), that the stump was nonfunctional and was not used (these are nonprosthesis cases). The opposite limb bore a double burden in that it received excessive use. The differences in sidedness were striking. On the side of the amputation not only the amputated bone remnant (upper arm bone or thigh bone) was atrophied in all respects, but also the bones of the associated limb-girdle (pelvis for the femur, clavicle (collarbone) and scapula (shoulder-blade) for the humerus).

It is of passing interest here to point out that the weightlessness of space flight, even though of short duration, causes a mild degree of bone demineralization, as determined by densitometric studies of X-ray films.

There is no doubt that exercise, involving functional use of muscle groups, has a stimulating effect on what I call "the functional growth picture." By this I mean growth of local bone tissue (sites of muscle attachment, cortical thickness, mineralization), growth of skeletal or voluntary muscle, and changes in body components as seen in breadths and girths, i.e., the skin-fat-muscle relationship shows a diminution of the fat component, an increase in the muscle-bone compartments.

It has been recently demonstrated in adults that exercise does in fact increase the outpouring of the growth hormone, except when carbohydrates are ingested during the exercise. The need for fuel as a result of the exercise is met by mobilization of stored body fat. The added growth hormone is largely responsible for starting and maintaining this source of fuel energy.

There are variables, especially in growing children, other than that of exercise. The age and physical condition of the child at the beginning of the exercise program must be considered. Consider too the body-build: a child of muscular build to begin with will but accentuate his build; a fat child will burn up some of the fat and gain some muscle; a very slender child will be helped, of course, but he won't end up with the "athletic" physique of the child well-built to begin with. Finally, type, intensity, and duration of the exercise must be fit into the end-result. Changes of short-term or irregular regimes of exercise are not lasting. About all one can say of them is that they are better than nothing at all.

During growth the total physical work capacity of the child shows no sex differences up to ten years of age, at which time males forge rapidly ahead. Work capacity gradually increases to twenty years, and then slowly decreases. There are no differences between white and Negro. In Philadelphia recently Rodahl of Lankenau Hospital found interesting regional differences within the urban area. The boys of North Philadelphia were superior to those of the same age of South Philadelphia in weight, height, muscle strength and work capacity. A finding such as this indicates that "norms" for physical variables in an urban population should be evaluated in terms of possible regional differences. As between North and South Philadelphia there are certain ethnic differences to be considered, plus possible socio-economic and nutritional factors. This type of analytic care is relevant to the diversified population subsamples of any urban area.

This leads to mention of race differences in motor and/ or athletic performance: Negro and white. Malina has surveyed the data in this area. At the elementary school level the Negro is a bit ahead in gross motor performance: one study showed him to perform better in a total of five motor tasks. Another showed that a higher per cent of Negro boys passed all of the Kraus-Weber motor performance battery at fourth-grade level. In test items designed by the American Association of Health, Physical Education, and Recreation, at fifth- and sixth-grade level,

Negro boys were superior in five of seven, Negro girls in four of seven. In Philadelphia elementary school children Malina found Negro boys and girls faster in running, but no racial differences in the standing broadjump or softball throw for distance. At high school and college level the Negro male exceeds in vertical jumping. One physical educator has summed it up: in eighty-one chances in one hundred Negro boys will surpass the white boys in "general athletic ability."

Racial differences in strength are not clearly established. Philadelphia Negro boys and girls age 6:0–12:0 years showed higher values in four measures of static strength. In another study Negro girls were found to be higher in grip strength by 2 kg. at 9:0–17:0 years; in boys the Negro had a higher score at 9:0–11:0 years, the white at 12:0–14:0 years.

Athletics

At this point I want to turn to organized exercise in the form of athletic participation. A participant, boy or girl, should have a good measure of fitness: 1) medical, or sound efficient body systems and organs; 2) functional, or a body efficient in the performance of strenuous work; 3) motor skills, or balanced muscle strength and coordination. There is an important statement to be made at this point: the judgment of fitness—indeed its very nature—is a function of maturation age rather than of chronological age. The early-maturing boy, age for age, is more ready (more "fit") than the late-maturing boy. I should like to see screening on this basis, particularly in the pre- and circumpubertal years (those of junior high and high school) when organized athletics takes the stage.

Studies at the University of California have shown that adolescent boys with good physical abilities are more muscular and sturdy in body-build, are more physically fit, are early maturing, are high in social prestige, and are better adjusted to the problems of their adolescent world.

On the contrary, boys with poor physical abilities are less muscular and slender in body build, are less physically fit ("poorer health"), are late maturing, are low in social prestige, and are poorly adjusted to the stresses of their adolescent world. It goes without saying that athletic potential should be tapped in the first group—they are the ones that can stand the gaff best. There is no reason, though, why an athletic program (ideally noncompetitive) should not be provided for the second group, but *scaled to levels of their competence and capacity.*

Growing children seem to have boundless energy. They also like group or gang participation and seem to feel the need for some kind of hobby or recreational outlet. Why not channel this energy, this peer-group appeal, this need for orientation to a goal, into a guided program of athletics? The result will be to train the child in endurance, strength, agility, flexibility of motor skills—*but* a program not only guided but adapted, I repeat, to *individual ability.*

As one who has researched child growth and development for over forty years I am wholeheartedly in favor of regular regimes of exercise, so that the growing body will have a better-balanced muscle-bone-tissue relationship. This I firmly believe and enthusiastically endorse. I also am on the side of those who would channel an exercise program into organized participation, i.e., various sport activities. This is all to the good. But if the organization of sports for children goes in the direction of *completely competitive activity,* then I register a vigorous protest, for then organization of the sport activity may spill over into the exploitation of the child. Here are some of the problems in this business of highly competitive sports:

1. By virtue of the maturation-age factor it is difficult to *match* competing individuals or teams.
2. There is a danger of *over-emphasis* (usually by non-participants, as alumni, townspeople, etc.), so that the youngsters may be impelled to excessive physical and emotional strain.

3. "*Winning* is the name of the game" is all too common a primary emphasis; "we gotta win this one fellows" is the type of exhortation that goes far beyond the idea of sport-for-sport's-sake, which I regard as basic.*
4. Far too often a total athletic program in a school is neglected by too great a concentration on *varsity sports*.

The growing child must be protected lest he overtax his growing body, either by total effort put out, by undue strain on a limb or joint, or by the hazards of jolting body contacts. Joint-strain is showing up in baseball, for the throwing arms, particularly in young pitchers, are manifesting elbow-joint problems, usually inflammatory, giving rise to a "pitcher's elbow" syndrome. This syndrome may go further than mere inflammation (osteochondritis), for it may involve trauma to the growth centers at the elbow: lower end of upper arm bone, upper ends of the forearm bones (radius and ulna).

Football

When I refer to "jolting body contacts" I can mean but one sport: football. Let's take a long, hard look at this competitive sport—but let me look with eyes of a professional growth researcher.

I am not interested in condemnation. That is biased and unscientific. I am interested in evaluation, to the best of my experience and my insight into growth problems. Hence, I propose to pursue two lines of thought: 1) offer certain evidence as to why football comes in for special scrutiny; 2) present certain hypotheses suggesting that the age-period under discussion is one of hyper-vulnerability, both physical and emotional.

---

*The idea of a game played solely to win may result in a terrific psychological effect, one of over-responsibility. Here is an example: in a bike test the individual was given two trial runs, the first to set his own pace, the second to "beat your own record." In the second run many failed and became nauseated, a psychosomatic reaction to what was thought of as a personal failure.

The Committee on Injuries and Fatalities for the American Football Coaches Association estimates that annually there are more than a million teen-agers playing football on sixteen thousand high school fields and sandlots. If so-called "peewee" and "midget" teams be included (often involving boys as young as eight, nine, or ten) I suppose another hundred thousand might well be added. Of the annual total mentioned by the Committee, about one in four will be hurt one way or another—sprains, bruises, lost teeth, and so on. Some eighty thousand of these injured boys will be hurt far more seriously —fractures, concussions, internal injuries. In one twenty-five year period, five hundred and eighteen football players have been killed, two hundred and ninety-three in high schools, one hundred and fifty-eight on sandlots; these last two add up to four hundred and fifty-one, or eighty-seven per cent of total deaths!

In 1965 the Statistical Bulletin of the Metropolitan Life Insurance Co. discussed "Hazards in Competitive Athletics."

Football accounted for ninety-five deaths in the United States during the five-year period, 1960–64, as shown in the table below:

Source	Direct	Indirect
College	12	7
High School	66	34
Pro and semi-pro	4	2
Sandlot	13	10
Totals	95	53

. . . Football contributes substantially to the annual toll of victims (in sports). According to data compiled by the American Football Coaches Association, 148 deaths were attributed to this sport in the past five years, two fifths more than in 1955–59. The tabulation shows fatal injuries due to activities directly associated with the game, such as blocking and tackling, increased about one fifth, deaths indirectly related to the game—such as those caused by heart failure, heat stroke, and other conditions—doubled.

The foregoing statistics are, in my opinion, enough to focus an inquiring spotlight on junior and even senior high school football—particularly the former.

In 1952 The Joint Committee on Athletic Competition for Children of Elementary and Junior High School Age reported on "Desirable Athletic Competition for Children." The basic age period covered was twelve to fifteen years. A total of two hundred and twenty physicians (pediatricians, cardiologists, orthopedists, physiologists, general practitioners) responded to a questionnaire concerning structural and functional factors influencing kind and extent of athletic activity. A summary follows:

	Affirmative	
Factor	*Number*	*Per cent*
Greater vulnerability of joints to injury (187)	85	45
Special hazard in connection with fractures of the epiphyseal area of long bones (187)	88	47
Disproportion of heart size to total body mass (177)	57	32
More likelihood for carry-over of activity past the stage of healthful fatigue to harmful exhaustion (177)	118	61
Greater susceptibility to rheumatic fever (177)	52	29
Greater difficulty determining the healthy heart as a prerequisite to activity (177)	53	30

(Numbers in parentheses refer to total answers for each factor)

If the per cents be averaged—and I'm not sure this is defensible—about forty per cent of the replies consider the factors, as a whole, of *positive value* in considering *any kind* of athletic activity.

Now, let's go a step onward. The same two hundred twenty physicians evaluated football on a four-fold basis:

1. Prohibited—Not advisable for this age group under any condition or plan.

   104 of 220 said yes. (*47%*)

2. Intramural—Sports program limited to contests between teams within individual school.

64 of 220 said yes. (*29%*)

3. Intramural and Invitational—Intramural sports ending in a few informal invitational games.

43 of 220 said yes. (*19%*)

4. Interschool—Sports program of varsity pattern including championship schedules.

22 of 220 said yes. (*10%*)

Nearly one-half are against any football in this age group; only one in ten favor the present intensively competitive set-up; about twenty-five per cent favor intramural competition.

As I pointed out earlier, we don't "just grow." There is nothing mechanical, nothing easy, about the process of circumpubertal growth. It is a wearing, tearing, all-consuming physiological process as far as organic balance is concerned. For here is the greatest energy turnover the body has known since the first year of life, or ever will know again. Here is the dramatic pulsating surge of growth and development that will make of the boy a man, of the girl, a woman. Here is, I insist, a growth period so dynamic, so dramatic, so resurgent, that its very nature renders it doubly vulnerable. What do I mean by this?

We grow—add to bone, muscle, organs—as the result of a heightened metabolic gradient known as anabolic, i.e., we add to body tissue at a speeded-up rate that results in a bigger body (bigger bones, bigger muscles, larger heart, lungs, intestines, etc.). This anabolic phase means, in simplest terms, that available bodily energy is directed mainly, almost solely, to the demands of organic growth. In the pre- and circumpubertal periods by far the greatest percentage of total available bodily energy (eighty per cent? ninety per cent?) is channeled into tissue building. The twenty per cent or ten per cent "left over" (in the total organism) is, in my opinion, far too precious to be directed (not to say wasted) in exercise demands that are, *at that period, exorbitant.*

Now, I may make clear what I mean by *"vulnerability."* I mean that in the terrific growth surge of the early teens the ratio between energy intake and energy output is nearly balanced or equated. What there is in excess had better be channeled into the less strenuous demands of curricular and social life. If this balance or equation be tipped in the direction of excessive functional demands— such as those inherent in the rough-and-tumble of football —then fatigue may cross the threshold of exhaustion, of depletion or near-depletion of physiological and nervous energy. That is what "vulnerability" means—it is a sort of energy-nakedness when growth and exercise demands are excessive.

The use of the term "nervous energy" focuses upon another aspect of the problem. If the early adolescent period be one of growth instability it is just as surely one of emotional tension and possible maladjustment. The period is one of awareness of self, realization of others, re-evaluation of one's whole world, especially at inter-personal level. The "moodiness," "dreaminess," "irrita-bility," "self consciousness" (to use but a few adjectives commonly describing the young adolescent) are but sur-face manifestations of deep-rooted tensions—not spiritual so much as physiological and biochemical. The very chemistry of the body is being resynthesized as never before and the essence of this ferment is distilled into behavioral reactions of many and varied sorts. Here, then, is another sphere of "vulnerability." If at this time foot-ball—or any game—be emphasized to the point where winning is an all-in-all (a zenith) and defeat an end-all (a nadir) then taut nerves and tensed tissues may vibrate to the point of "breaking." Thus the problem shapes into a psychosomatic one.

The growing human body is a wonderfully integrated mechanism. As it matures step by step (literally and fig-uratively), it becomes an increasingly useful body, a faithful servant of the individual. All those who serve the growing child—parents, school personnel, the medical profession, the total community—should see that he gets every chance for healthy, normal growth, and effective, dynamic bodily well-being.

XI

GROWING BODY AND DEVELOPING BEHAVIOR

Behavior Beginning: Organic

In a sense this chapter will focus on the body-mind problem—and it *is* a problem!

> What is Mind?
> No matter!
>
> What is Matter?
> Never mind!

The *body* is organic, but the *mind* (as contrasted with the brain) is supra-organic. Yet the mind is in and of the brain, and the mind is related to *all* behavior as a mediator or conditioner. In this sense, therefore, behavior is the sum total of the interaction between the biologico-physiological organism and its environment. Behavior is, with growth, increasingly adaptive, as the child learns patterns of socially acceptable behavior. So, behavior becomes bio-cultural.

Behavior pattern in the child, in an organic sense, is prenatal and is well organized before birth. At the seventh-eighth fetal (lunar) month movements are vague, there is little or no muscle tone, breathing is shallow, sucking and swallow reflexes are slight, the cry and grasp are weak, the light reflex is slight, and when the fetus is prone he can turn his head. At the eighth-ninth fetal (lunar) month movements are purposive, muscle tone is fair, the startle reflex is present, there are periods of wakefulness, the grasp is strong, the hunger cry is good, and when the fetus is prone he turns his head and elevates his rump. At the ninth-tenth fetal (lunar) month movements are vigorous, muscle tone is good, he may "track" with his eyes, the startle reflex is very strong, the cry is vigorous, there is response to a caress, hands "make a good fist," the sucking-swallowing reflexes are strong, and when the fetus is prone he may try to lift his head.

Not only is organic behavior (neuromuscular) prenatal but its developmental patterning is prehuman. Studies have shown that when body-movement patterns (limb/head movements) and locomotor patterns (sitting, creeping, bipedal standing, bipedal walking) are compared for chimpanzee and man the rank-order correlation is $+0.88$; in other words both the baby chimp and human baby develop body-use and walking behavior in nearly an identical fashion. Moreover, the chimp achieves the same motor behavior level when his brain is 49.6% of its adult weight, as when the child's brain is 51.7% of its adult weight.

So much for the development of organic (motor) behavior, both human and comparative. Is there any evidence that there is a relationship between the organic self and the psycho-social self? To put the question directly: is fetal activity related, possibly, to postnatal personality development? Sontag, of the Fels Research Institute, presents some suggestive research data. Two terms are defined here: *psychosomatic* describes the "physiological disturbance associated with modified autonomic [involuntary] nervous system function, emotional in origin"; *somatopsychic* describes how the "basic physiological processes affect personality structure, perception, and performance of the individual."

The fetal activity of twenty-four males was observed during the last three months of pregnancy: quick-kicking movements, rhythmic turning of the body, and fetal hiccoughs; also observed was the fetal heart-rate in ten-beat segments over a period of five to ten minutes. A number of observations were made on the mother, e.g., her nutrition, activities, nitrogen balance, emotional state, cigarette-use, and so on. At two years of age the child was placed in the nursery school for a two-week period of observation and testing (some tests had started at six months, others were introduced, and were continued). Home visits were made until age eight, and parent interviews were begun then. From six to eighteen years a number of tests measuring autonomic stress were given.

A pattern of response defined as "social apprehension" was recognized: hesitancy in joining groups; anxiety in the face of threatened peer aggression; reluctance to enter the nursery school car (to leave the home). The more active fetus was much more likely to be socially apprehensive (a culturo-behavioral "scaredy-cat") at 2:6 years; the heart-beat showed sudden bursts of rate-acceleration. Sontag called this total picture *cardiac lability-stability*. He concluded that the level of dependency was significantly greater in cardiac labiles from the fetal period to age eighteen years: they are reluctant to depend on love objects; they have more conflicts over dependency; they have a more intense striving for achievement, and greater anxiety over erotic behavior; they are more introspective and are vacillatory in decision-making.

Evidence of this sort leads one to conclude that there must be an organic substrate to the expression of behavior. The problem is not one of absolute determinism but one of relative mediation. Body doesn't make behavior, but it does influence it in many rather intangible ways. Body-mind (brain) are there to influence, and to be influenced by, the environment.

At birth the baby can see, hear, and smell, but he cannot taste discriminatively. He is sensitive to touch, pain, and change of position. When he is two hours old his pupils dilate in the dark, constrict in light, and he can follow a fast-moving light with his eyes. He can smack his lips, suck or chew his fingers or suck a nipple in his mouth, and if the corner of his mouth or cheek is touched he will turn to the side, right or left, of the stimulation. In terms of total body movement he can lift his chin from a prone position, react to a loud sound with his entire body, flex and extend his limbs, grasp an object placed in his palm, and he can cry, cough, vomit, or turn away.

In larger sense the newborn finds himself in a world of hunger, of pain, and of variation in hot/cold circumstances. He learns almost at once that he can somehow play a part in an environmental conditioning: he can participate in, and even formulate, patterns of stimulus-response at mother-child level. In effect *he is now a social being.* He is soon aware that the irritable or protesting babe—more often male than female—gets more maternal attention. The child's whole first year sees a rapid development in his perceptual structuring.

As I have studied physical growth and behavior in the child I have never ceased to marvel at the incredible capacity of the human brain (human mind) which permits and facilitates human behavior with all of its capabilities and potentials.

Lassek, a neurologist, has figured out what would be needed to *construct* a human brain: one and a half million cubic feet of space, one million kilowatts of electric power, one billion trillion each of wires and miniature tubes, at a cost of two million trillion dollars! And all this would only "crudely simulate the human brain from a physiological viewpoint." In our brain, our central nervous system, there are twenty billion neurons which we run on only twenty-five watts of electric power. It is estimated that we use only one to ten per cent of our brain potential at any one time.

In 1543 Andreas Vesalius, an anatomist, said, "How the brain performs its functions in imagination, in reasoning, in thinking, and in memory, I can form no opinion whatever." Today, four hundred and twenty-seven years later, we're at about the same level of perplexity—although the computer-brain comparison gives a little better insight into the input-output situation.

The Five Ages of the Child

Shakespeare has immortalized the seven ages of a man. In essence these seven ages are an incisive categorization of the way-stations on the journey through life.

I want now to call attention to the five ages of childhood, literally from conception to the twentieth year of postnatal life, but I shall consider the birth to twenty year period. I have already mentioned the more purely biological ages, but I shall repeat them here and tie them in with several nonbiological ages, or behavioral ages:

I. *Chronological Age* (C.A.): this is the birthday or calendric-age of the child. It is based on sidereal time and is constant, i.e., *all* children born on July 1, 1961 are ten years old on July 1, 1971.

II. *Biologic or Organic Age:* this is the registry of the rate of progress toward maturity (sexual, adult). It is a variable age, and has several sub-categories:

   1. *Morphological Age:* this is the relation of attained size to normative size. For example, a child may have a Height Age (H.A.) of eight years, even though his C.A. is ten years. This means that at C.A. of ten he has the height equivalent of a boy of C.A. of eight, i.e., he is short for his age. It is variable, with tall, mid, and short family-lines.

   2. *Skeletal Age* (S.A.): this is the registry of biologic

time in the developing skeleton, as assessed from a wrist-hand X-ray film. It is variable, with early, mid, and late maturer categories.

3. *Dental Age* (D.A.): this is the variable to moderately variable registry of biologic time in the developing dentition. There are two main categories of D.A.:

   a. Calcification Age: the stage-sequence of tooth development from first appearance of cusp(s) to root apical closure.

   b. Eruption Age: the progressive emergence of the tooth from its alveolus or socket into functional occlusion.

4. *Circumpubertal Age:* this is the variable of primary and secondary sexual maturity. In terms of growth-timing its import is in its growth velocity: it is the time of the oft-called adolescent spurt, or circumpubertal acceleration in growth.

III. *Behavioral or Emotional:* this is a measure, of increasing variability and complexity, of the child's progressive adaptation to, and indoctrination in, the cultural milieu of which he is a part. In essence this is the total socialization process.

IV. *Intellectual or Mental Age:* this is the variable and very complex measure of the child's realization of cerebral or mental potential. This involves the total learning situation of the child. There is here involved the factor of intelligence, however it be measured.

V. *The Self-Concept Age:* this is often overlooked but it is extremely basic to the child's ego-development. This is the way the child perceives self (the mirror-image in true sense) as a conformist, or non-conformist, in physical growth, in time and rate of maturation, and in behavioral patterning. Basically this is a fluctuant age, for it often varies *within* an individual life.

Learning

Jean Piaget, the great French student of child behavior, recognizes four major phases in learning: 1) birth to two years; 2) two to seven years; 3) seven to eleven years; 4) eleven to fifteen years.

The first period is called the "trial-and-error logic" of infancy and is essentially pragmatic—what succeeds is adopted, what fails is rejected.

In the second the child is basically self-oriented, not necessarily selfishly so, but more in terms of own ego. He learns that actions have causes—*and* have effects! He is intellectually immature in this midchildhood, and this immaturity must not be interpreted as perversity. Essentially this is the I-want-to-know-*why* time of behavioral development.

The third period is one of behavioral status quo (and, interestingly enough, a quiescent time in physical growth also). The environment is regulated as best it can be in terms of the habitual, the usual, the unchanged. Behavioral security is thus achieved, anchored in a veritable sea of tranquility. The threshold of logic is often reached at the end of this period.

The fourth period brings reasoning and the testing of observed facts. Alternative explanations are envisioned and abstractions and symbols are incorporated into patterns of thinking and doing.

The entire process of understanding—of learning—says Piaget, is a function of the rate of maturation of mental powers, and these powers must be reinforced by regular and continuous use. The stage-by-stage learning process, he avers, is the coming to maturity of genetically entrenched potentials, i.e., learning involves both inherent capacities and the environmental stimuli of the educational process.

There is every reason to believe in the over-all oneness

of an integrated pattern of biological and behavioral unfolding, which may be expressed as follows:

Growth (dimensional change)

+

Maturation (structural-functional change)
(lead to)

↓

Changes in performance possibilities
(which lead to)

↓

Stages of *readiness*
(which lead to)

↓

Integrative functioning
(which is)

↓

Learning (an increase in adequacy of function
via repetitive practice of the function)
(which leads to)

↓

The concept of *Developmental Task* (a blend
between a biological need and a societal
demand)

This is to say that there is a bio-cultural continuum, that there is synchrony in total growth, that there is a correlation between the physically growing child and the behaviorally developing child, and, moreover, that there are intercorrelations *within* the biological spheres and *within* the behavioral areas.

Relation of Size and Maturation to the IQ

The problem of the relation of the body to behavior has centered around two main dimensions; 1) size, usually as expressed by body height; and 2) maturation, as expressed by skeletal development. It goes without saying that growth and maturation of the brain is certainly a prepotent factor: at birth the brain has twenty-five per cent of its adult weight, at six months fifty per cent, at two and a half years seventy-five percent, at five years ninety per cent, and at seven plus years ninety-five per cent plus. Most often the behavioral trait selected for comparison with a body trait is in the intellectual area as measured by the I.Q.

In 1968, Churchill and associates studied fifty-one school-age children with "undifferentiated" mental retardation, who had significantly lower birth weight than fifty-one control children with I.Q.'s of 110+. The two groups were matched for sex, age, and socio-economic status in the same middle-class segment of the population (Detroit). There was a positive correlation between birth weight and the I.Q. even when birth weights below 2,500 gms and gestation ages under 38 weeks were eliminated. It is hypothesized that brain maturation and birth weight were both inhibited if the intra-uterine nourishment were inadequate.

At the Fels Research Institute, Kagan and Garn reported a correlation between body-build and the I.Q. Children of LL (large chested) and SS (small chested) parents were studied. The LL and SS children were sorted out and it was found that the LL's had a significantly higher I.Q. at two-three-three and a half years, but from four to ten years the differences were negligible. Then the child's own chest was scored at age two years and used as a predictor. The L-chested boys did significantly better in perceptual motor and language development tests than did the S-chested from three to six years. The L- or S-chest relationship with the I.Q. was not found in girls. It is suggested (perhaps because the child already has learned to use larger size confidently?) that a large bony chest diameter "is associated with a less fearful approach to problem situations."

In 1893 a pediatrician named Porter looked at St. Louis school children and their test grades. He found that at any given age pupils with higher test scores were bigger (taller and heavier). Ergo, he said, physical growth is related to mental growth. In 1895 Franz Boas, an anthropologist, said "nonsense"—all that was proved was that the two growths (physical and mental) tend to go together, not that the one depends on the other. For Worcester, Mass., school children he showed that size (height) differences are due to variations in the tempo (rate or speed) of growth:

	Grades			
Chronological Age	**1**	**2**	**3**	**4**
7 years	6.9*	7.8	7.9	—
8 years	7.7	8.3	8.9	9.5
9 years	—	9.0	9.4	9.7

(*these are height ages, i.e. Grade 1 has a height age range of 6.9–7.7 years, Grade 2 one of 7.8–9.0 years, and so on)

In 1941 Boas studied the relations between height age, weight age, and maturational age, referred to the I.Q. He found a significant regression of the I.Q. on height and maturation ages at a given chronological age. He concluded that "the close correlation between anatomical and psychological traits in childhood must be interpreted as due to the influence of the tempo of physiological development over the body and its functions." It seemed logical for him to conclude that differences in rates of maturing occur in mental ability as well as in size as represented by height and weight. This does not prove, however, that there is co-advancement, namely that the rates in physical and mental growth accelerate at the same time.

Recent studies have shown that while there is a positive correlation between various psychological tests and stature, the correlation is high enough to suggest size as a factor—one of many—but it is not high enough to be predictive. If a bright seventh-grader is taller than his peers he is not necessarily bright because he's tall; he may be *both* tall *and* bright because he is maturationally advanced. Then again, he may be tall because he had tall parents and bright because of high familial and personal motivation.

There is another factor that I should like to suggest: people often react to a child large for age as though he were more "mature" in the sense that more can be expected of him. I speak from experience. I am 6'4½" tall and was tall as a child (literally head and shoulders over my age-peers). I remember that, grade for grade, the teacher singled me out for chores demanding not only strength but responsibility. In a very real way this meant that my size was an evocative factor: more was expected and demanded of me. My responses to this made, I am sure, for an accelerated pace in my development of certain personality traits, as "dependability," "willingness," "ability," and so on.

The relation between tallness and high-scoring and possibly advanced height and advanced test is not purely morphological alone, i.e., height alone. Size *is* a factor, I'm sure, but not for itself alone. There are two things to consider: 1) size and maturation often go hand-in-hand, for the early maturer is taller; hence size *plus* maturity in all probability play a dual role in the high-scorers; 2) the combination of size and maturity play an important psychological role, not only with reference to the individual (his self-concept of "taller," "more mature"), but also with reference to sex- and peer-groupings.

In 1963 Eichorn of the Institute of Child Welfare of the University of California studied the psycho-social behavior patterns of early and late maturing boys and girls. Grades H6–L7 through H9–L10 were studied semiannually, while Grades H10–L11 and H11–L12 were studied annually. This gave nine ratings over a six-year period (H = high, L = low).

Early maturing children, boys especially, are more self-confident and play a more mature social role; they provide the leaders in the various school activities; they score higher in such traits as attractiveness of physique, good appearance, grooming, matter-of-factness, unaffectedness, relaxation, popularity, leadership, humor regarding themselves, and having older friends.

Late maturers are more apt to feel personally inadequate, to have strong feelings of rejection and domination by others; they have prolonged dependency needs and often have a rebellious attitude toward parents; they score higher in such traits as attention-getting, eagerness, animation, uninhibitiveness, restlessness, talkativeness, bossiness, and self-assurance in class to the point of "being cocky."

It seems to me that what has been said up to now points strongly to the conclusion that much of human behavior—especially in the formative years—is a function not of morphology, per se, but the way in which the total environment supports and facilitates behavior development, and the way in which morphology is reacted to (and demands made of it) by self and by peers.

Genetics and the I.Q.

In Chapter IX the role of heredity in morphology has been discussed. What about behavior, including intelligence? The answer seems to be that there is a hereditary component in many aspects of intellectual developing. For example, twin studies have demonstrated a highly significant correlation of between-twin I.Q.: almost the same in identical twins reared together, less, though still very high, in identical twins reared apart; moderately high, but much higher than for siblings, in fraternal twins reared together. In a recent survey of human behavior genetics Vandenberg (1969) notes a hereditary component in the following learning traits (listed in decreasing order of strength of the component): word fluency, verbal facility (including spelling and grammar), spatial ability, clerical speed and accuracy, reasoning, number ability, and memory.

Then, almost ambivalently, we look once more at the parent-child relationship. The parent-child correlation for boys and girls is significantly high when three parental variables are evaluated, i.e., an index of parental ability, traits (especially maternal) associated with learning in the child, and emotional support by the parents. Thus it is possible to predict about fifty per cent of the variance of a child's performance ability at age eighteen if the parental traits in the child's preschool years are known and properly weighted. The chances are that this environmental nurture affords a better prediction of intelligence at adolescence than does the child's own I.Q. score at three years of age.

The parent-child relation with the child's I.Q. at three, six, and ten years has been studied by University of California psychologists. Parental education level was ascertained and the parental I.Q. was determined. Maternal education correlated higher than paternal education with boys and girls at all three ages; also, the maternal education was a better predictor of the girls' I.Q. than of the boys' I.Q. at all three ages. Finally, the maternal "drive" or pressure toward the child played a big role in determining the child's I.Q.

There is an early-manifested sex difference in the development of behavior patterns. In studies of preschool children at the Fels Institute it has been found that girls were behaviorally advanced in the ninety-one items of the Gesell test: item by item the girls passed earlier in the entire ninety-one, and scored higher in sixty-one of the ninety-one. This sex difference was matched by a corresponding advancement in maturation rate and age. Girls were ahead, often by ten per cent plus in *all* seventeen language items (speaking words, naming, waving "bye-bye," etc.). In general motor behavior the difference was less, but in perceptual motor ability the boys were ahead (form-board, performance box, triangle-drawing, circle-copying, rod-in-hole activity, etc.). In all the tests sister-sister similarity was much greater than brother-brother or sister-brother.

Readiness

Physical growth has many stages or optimum times for structural and functional (behavioral) advancement. In essence these stages or times represent a functional capacity or potentiality which may be termed readiness. There are a series of "best times" in the developmental progress of the growing child when a level of expectancy may be translated into performance. There are many such "best times"—for neuromuscular coordination, for training and cultural indoctrination, and so forth. There are also "best times" for learning and the entire complexity of the educative process. Readiness is not an abstraction: rather it is specific and it is task-oriented, i.e., it is directed to the performance of a demand, be that demand reading, writing, spelling, arithmetic or any other chore in the school set-up. Readiness is, therefore, a functional inter-relationship between the ability of the child and the school demands.

Here is a sequence that sets the stage: with growth and maturation—wherein form, function, and biological time proceed synchronously—there is a series of progressive function possibilities. This may be termed over-all behavioral readiness, from which develop patterns of performance in terms of integrated functioning. These patterns are sequentially time-linked and as they emerge they are integrated with changes in function and performance. The entire organism is involved in the learning process. This process is covert (innate) and overt (assigned societal and cultural tasks).

Brenner (1957) states that three fundamental requisites in readiness are:

1. subject-object orientation   S ⟷ O
2. individual-task directedness   I ⟷ T
3. individual-goal directedness   I ⟷ G

Essentially school success or failure of a child depends upon an ability-task load balance or ratio. If ability is too low or task-load too high there is trouble. Here is Brenner's scheme (IV = individual volume, TV = task volume):

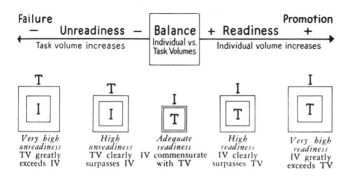

Failure				Promotion
— Unreadiness —		Balance	+ Readiness +	
Task volume increases		Individual vs. Task Volumes	Individual volume increases	

Very high unreadiness TV greatly exceeds IV | *High unreadiness* TV clearly surpasses IV | *Adequate readiness* IV commensurate with TV | *High readiness* IV clearly surpasses TV | *Very high readiness* IV greatly exceeds TV

A scheme such as this is a working hypothesis and not much more. What it does is to provide a framework of evaluation involving the parent→ child ←teacher relationship. Note that the arrows in this triad both point to the child. The TV may exceed the IV for a number of reasons; such as an innately low IV due to lowered I.Q., poor health, malnutrition, poor home environment, and so on; the TV may be too high-scaled for the cultural or the socio-economic milieu of the individual. The IV-TV imbalances can be ascertained in the school and evaluated by parent *plus* teacher. It is too often the "Establishment" —the School—that takes the blame when the home environment, in toto, is at fault.

Certainly I have no universal panacea for the IV–TV school confrontation, save, as a biologist, to point out that IV *does* relate to maturation level. Mayhap TV should be adjusted to the "shorn lamb," in this case the late maturer, for in his case TV is *relatively* too large, whereas for all others it is *absolutely* too small. At all grade levels there are those who struggle, those for whom "it's a breeze!"

Growth—Behavior Patterns

To illustrate what I believe to be an over-all concordance between physical growth and behavioral development I present two major themes: Patterns of Physical Growth and The Unfolding Personality. Each will be presented in identical five chronological age-periods. Therefore, the physical items (emphasizing body use) in Early Childhood and the personality items, also in Early Childhood are—as sets of items—more or less synchronously emergent. This is true of all growth-periods. One other word: the order of the items a, b, c, d . . . is not an absolute. The sequence is my idea of importance, not necessarily the order of appearance.

PATTERNS OF PHYSICAL GROWTH

i. *Early Childhood* (3–6 years)
   a. Posture habits begin; trunk-limb coordination basic.
   b. Promote uniform growth of muscular, skeletal, and organ systems.
   c. Exercise should stress arms, shoulder, upper body.
   d. Precision in movement is goal, with skill later; stress running, climbing ropes, bars, etc.; simple play activity.
   e. Coordination basic, with strength, speed, agility not stressed.
ii. *Middle Childhood* (6–9 years)
   a. Posture important and exercise must emphasize this.

b. Smoothness, sureness, and body-use skills progress.

c. Muscle strength important, especially by nine years.

d. Boys focus on self-testing "stunts."

e. Group games and rhythmics useful at this stage.

III. *Late Childhood* (9–11 years)

a. Balance, agility, endurance, power stressed.

b. Improvement of earlier-learned skills plus new, more specialized skills.

c. Development of strength important.

d. Organized team games begin, but stress individual athletics.

e. Personal performance very important.

IV. *Early Adolescence* (girls 10–12 years, boys 11–14 years)

a. Attention paid to strength, power, flexibility, speed, agility.

b. No new skills; improvement of earlier skills.

c. Organized sports, but must not involve excessive strain on heart, joints, muscles.

V. *Late Adolescence* (girls 12–16 years, boys 14–18 years)

a. Physical conditioning of major importance.

b. Individual potentiality is goal, facilitated by individual sports.

c. But team-sport is still important.

d. Boys stress power, girls grace and personal attractiveness.

THE UNFOLDING PERSONALITY

I. *Early Childhood* (3–6 years)

a. Strong need for affection and for parents to be demonstrative in concern and affection.

b. Security need in approval and assigned tasks; discipline should be consistent, meaningful.

c. Great self-interests; questions of own origin.

d. Need for companionship; boy-girl play should not have a "rough" vs. "delicate" sex emphasis.

e. Sex organ manipulation common as mere curiosity.

II. *Middle Childhood* (6–9 years)

    a. More independent, but still need for security via adult approval.

    b. Take selves seriously; resent adult "butting in."

    c. Frequent use of vulgar words; antisocial attitudes relate to wearing old clothes and fussing over personal cleanliness.

    d. Group interest, though unorganized; "gang" stage by nine years or so.

    e. Fear of things not understood; may include physician, dentist, hospital.

    f. Sexual modesty at nine years ($\pm$); still prefer own sex; sex interest mild if earlier questions answered objectively.

III. *Late Childhood* (9–11 years)

    a. Earlier affection ties go; new period of "crushes" and hero-worship.

    b. Easily offended and "feels misunderstood."

    c. Very restless; childhood values of approval by adults disintegrate.

    d. Peer pattern basic to group approval: cliques, clubs, "secret societies," etc.; hates to be "chicken."

    e. Day-dreams common; type of fantasy may produce guilt feeling.

    f. Sexes still tend to keep self-consciously separate.

IV. *Early Adolescence* (girls 10–12 years, boys 11–14 years)

    a. Phenomenon of puberty often accompanied by psychosomatic emotional instability centering around variation in time, acne, perspiration-odor, etc.

    b. Group approval paramount in terms recognition and attention.

    c. Demand for privacy; often excessive modesty; guilt-complex over masturbation.

    d. Excessive activity or eating may mask feeling of insecurity.

    e. Girls socialize earlier; "crushes" frequent but of short duration.

    f. Physical contact of sexes via dancing, both folk- and social dancing.

  v. *Late Adolescence* (girls 12–16 years, boys 14–18 years)

    a. Group status basic with respect both to physique and appearance; "rather be dead than different."

    b. If there is peer- or sex-group insecurity, the individual may take it out on parents; feelings intense.

    c. Revolt against parental authority (the "generation gap"); want adult privileges; this may be worsened by parental or family maladjustment.

    d. Girls always interested in boys and boys apt to be variable about girls; girls "fall in love" with older boys, boys with younger girls; need for physical contact in holding of hands, petting.

The foregoing listing of physical and behavioral traits is, I am well aware, not one hundred per cent exhaustive. I have indicated those traits and trait-complexes which in my experience, and from the literature, have seemed the most meaningful. Moreover, each is to a greater or less degree psychosomatic, partaking of the soma—the body— and of the psyche—the spirit; or, I dare say, of the quantity and quality of *Child Growth.*

There is much to-do these days about the "generation gap," vociferously asserted by the present younger generation. It may exist in terms of performance with respect to certain politico-socio-cultural problems, but I am not so sure that it exists in terms of awareness and perceptive understanding. The major difference seems to be between the younger "do-it-now" and the older "it-takes-a-bit-of-time" frames of mind. For an action program there must be a sense of dedication in *all;* young and old, working together and with each respecting the rights and needs of the other.

APPENDIX I

Some Statistical Tools

One often hears it said that "he's of *average* stature." The term "average" refers to a mean value of, say, twenty-five ten-year-old boys: the height of each is measured, the twenty-five heights are added up, and the resultant sum is divided by twenty-five (the number measured). The term "mean value" is synonymous with "average value."

Another statement often heard is, "he's not average, but he's in the *normal range of variation.*" This is a statistical device called "the standard deviation," which is calculated from the variations—in height, for example—in a given sample. Take again the sample of twenty-five boys above mentioned and let us say they have an average height of 58″ with a standard deviation (S.D.) of 2″. The S.D. is so calculated that sixty-seven per cent of all ten-year-old boys will range between 58″ minus 2″ and 58″ plus 2″, or 56″–60″. This is the mean (M) $\pm$ 1 S.D. This is the usually acceptable expression of a wholly acceptable range of variation. The range can be extended to M $\pm$ 2 S.D., and include ninety-five per cent of the entire sample: 58″ minus 4″ and 58″ plus 4″, or 54″–62″. The boy at 54″ is very short for 10 years, and the boy at 62″ is very tall for this age. Once more, this is an acceptable range to give an idea of extreme limits of normalcy.

The method most widely used by pediatricians is that of *percentile ranking*, which is easily determined by referral to percentile graphs. A ten-year-old boy may be ranked in stature as at the fifth percentile or at the ninety-fifth percentile: the first boy is very short, the second boy is very tall, or to put it another way, the first boy is in the *shortest* five in one hundred and the second boy is in the *tallest* five in one hundred. The "average" boy is at the fiftieth percentile.

Finally, in growth studies it is important to express degrees or amounts of relationship between two variables. We want to quantify, for example, how height and age are related during the child's growth. This is expressed as the *coefficient of correlation,* or Pearsonian r (after Karl Pearson, the English biometrician who developed the statistic). As the child gets older he gets taller; therefore, the correlation is *positive* ($r =$ about $+.80$). The adult gets older, but he does not get taller, so that r will be zero. In extreme old age he may get shorter due to loss of muscle tonus, and so on (he "shrinks" a bit) and the r will be negative. In general, in child growth, an r greater than $+0.35$ may be regarded as showing a significant correlation, i.e., the variables contrasted vary with respect to one another other than by random chance.

Author	Birth	1	2	3	4	5	6	7	8	9	10	11	12	13	14	15	16	17	18	19	20
Vierordt	Suckling B–1 yr.	Childhood: B–7 years							Boyhood: 7–14 years							Adolescence: 14 yrs. +					
		Deciduous teeth: 1–7 years							Permanent teeth: 7 years plus					Pubertal changes						
Stratz	Suckling: B–1½ years	Neutral age: 1½–7 yrs. First fill-out; First stretch; 1½–4 yrs.						Bisexual child: 7–15 years 2nd fill-out; 7–10 yrs.			2nd stretch; 10–15 yrs.						Puberty: 15 yrs. to maturity				
Bardeen	Infancy B–1½ yr.	Childhood: ½ yr. to puberty (ca. 13 years)												Adolescence: puberty to maturity (ca. 13 yrs.–ca. 20 yrs.)						
Bean	Infancy B–1 yr.	Childhood											*Prepubertal:*		*Puberty:*		*Adolescence:*					
		Milk teeth: 1–6 yrs.					Permanent teeth: 6–10 yrs.				10–12 yrs.		2-yr. period betw. 12–17 yrs.			3-yr. period after puberty				
Gray	Infancy: B–3 yrs.			Pre-school 3–6 yrs.			School period (slow growth) 6–12 yrs.						Puberty: approx. 12–15 yrs.			Late youth: 15–19 or 20 yrs.					
Heimendinger	Infant	I DECADE														II DECADE							
		Brain growth to 7 decid. teeth:– perm. teeth up to M2 Final deceleration: M3 eruption																				
	Suckling B–1 yr.	Pre-school: neural type Small child Play age					School: Lymphatic type Larger child														
													Puberty ♀ 11–13; ♂ 13–15			Adolescence ♂ 15–18; ♀ 13–16						
Krogman	B–1 yr.	♂ 1–16 ♀ 1–15 ← Childhood → (Puberty) ♂ 13–14 ♀ 13–14												Adolescence								
		Early 1–6				Mid 6 to 9–10			Late ♂ 9–10 to 16 ♀ 9–10 to 15			Late ♀ 12–13; ♂ 12–13		♂ 14 to 18–20 ♀ 13 to 18–20							

REFERENCES

Books

Arey, L. B. *Developmental Anatomy* (ed. 6). Philadelphia, 1954.

Bayer, L. M. and Bayley, N. *Growth Diagnosis*. Chicago, 1959.

Bayley, N. and Tuddenham, R. D. "Adolescent Changes in Body Build" (pp. 33–55 in *Adolescence*, ed. by N. B. Henry). Chicago, 1944.

Clarke, H. H. *Application of Measurement to Health and Physical Education* (ed. 4). Englewood Cliffs, N.J., 1967.

Drillien, C. M. *The Growth of the Prematurely Born Child*. London, 1964.

Drillien, C. M., Ingram, T. S. and Wilkinson, E. M. *The Causes and Natural History of Cleft Lip and Palate*. Baltimore, 1966.

Falkner, Frank (ed.). *Human Development*. Philadelphia, 1966.

Gardner, L. I. (ed.). *Endocrine and Genetic Diseases of Childhood*. Philadelphia, 1969.

Greulich, W. W. and Pyle, S. I. *Radiographic Atlas of Skeletal Development of the Hand and Wrist*. Stanford, 1959.

Hammons, H. G. (ed.). *Heredity Counselling* (see "Genetics in relation to cardiovascular diseases," pp. 42–56, by V. A. McKusick). New York, 1959.

Harris, H. A. *et al.* "The Measurement of Man." Minneapolis, 1930.

Harrison, G. A., Weiner, J. S., Tanner, J. M., Barnicot, N. A. *Human Biology*. New York, 1964.

Henry, N. B. (ed.). *Adolescence*. 43rd Yrbk. *Nat. Soc. Study Educ.*, Chicago, 1944.

Illingworth, R. S. *The Development of the Infant and Young Child: Normal and Abnormal*. London, 1967.

Krogman, W. M. *The Growth of Man.* Tabulae Biologicae, Vol. XX, pp. 962. The Hague, 1941.

Lassek, A. M. *The Human Brain.* Springfield, Ill., 1957.

Lipsitt, L. P. and Spiker, C. C. (eds.). *Advances in Child Development and Behavior* (Vol. 1). New York, 1963.

Martin, F. A. *Roberts' Nutrition Work with Children.* Chicago, 1954.

Scheinfeld, A. *Your Heredity and Environment.* Philadelphia, 1965.

Scrimshaw, N. S. and Gordon, J. E. (eds.). *Malnutrition, Learning, and Behavior.* Cambridge, Mass., 1968.

Shock, N. W. "Physiological Changes in Adolescence" (pp. 56–79 in *Adolescence,* ed. Henry, W. B.). Chicago, 1944.

Tanner, J. M. *Growth at Adolescence* (ed. 2). Oxford, 1962.

Tanner, J. M. *Human Growth.* New York, 1960.

Tanner, J. M., Taylor, G. R. and Editors of *Life. Growth.* New York, 1965.

Vandenberg, S. G. (ed.). *Progress in Human Behavior Genetics.* Baltimore, 1968.

Watson, E. H. and Lowrey, G. H. *Growth and Development of Children* (5th ed.). Chicago, 1967.

Williams, P. L. and Wendell-Smith, C. P. *Basic Human Embryology.* Philadelphia, 1966.

Monographs or Journals

Anderson, M., Green, W. T., and Messner, M. B. "Growth and Predictions of Growth in the Lower Extremities," in *J. Bone Joint Surg.* 45 A (1): 1–15, 1963.

Bayley, N. "Individual Patterns of Development," in *Child Development* 27 (1): 45–74. 1956.

Bayley, N. and Davis, F. C. "Growth Changes in Body Size and Proportions During the First Three Years: a Developmental Study of 61 Children by Repeated Measurements," in *Biometrika,* Vol. 27, Pts. I-II, pp. 26–87. 1931. u.c.

Bayley, N. and Pinneau, S. R. "Tables for Predicting Adult Height from Skeletal Age: Revised for Use with the Greulich-Pyle Hand Standards," in *J. Pediatrics.* 46(4): 423–441. 1952.

Biller, H. B. "Masculine Development: an Integrated Review," in *Merrill-Palmer Quarterly,* 12(4): 253–294. Oct., 1967.

Boas, F. "The Relation Between Physical and Mental Development," in *Science* 93: 339–342. 1941.

Brenner, A. "Nature and Meaning of Readiness for School," in *Merrill-Palmer Quarterly,* 3(3): 113–135. 1957.

Dahlberg, G. "An Explanation of Twins," in *Sci. Amer.* Jan. 1951.

Dean, R. T. A. "The Effects of Malnutrition on the Growth of Young Children" (pp. 111–122 in *Modern Problems in Pediatrics*, ed. by F. Falkner). Karger, N.Y., 1960.

Eichorn, D. "Biological Correlates of Behavior," in *62nd Yrbk. Nat. Soc. Study Educ.* Part I, Psychology. 61 pp. Chicago, 1963.

Falkner, F. *et al.* "Some International Comparisons of Physical Growth in the First Two Years of Life," in *Courier* (Paris). 8(1): 1–11. 1958.

Garn, S. M., Rohmann, C. G., and Silverman, F. N. "Radiographic Standards for Postnatal Ossification and Tooth Calcification," in *Med. Radiography and Photography* 41 (2): 45–65. 1967 (Eastman Kodak Co., Rochester, N.Y.).

Garn, S. M., Silverman, F. M., Hertzog, K. P. and Rohmann, C. G. "Lines and Bands of Increased Density: Implications to Growth and Development." *Med. Radiography and Photography*, 44 (3): 58–89. 1968 (Eastman Kodak Co., Rochester, N.Y.).

Graham, G. G. *et. al.* "Programs for Combatting Malnutrition in the Pre-school Child in Peru" (p. 163 ff. in *Pre-school Child Malnutrition: Primary Deterrant in Human Progress*. Nat. Acad. Sci. Washington, D.C., 1966.

Greulich, W. W. *et. al.* "Somatic and Endocrine Studies of Puberal Adolescent Boys," in *Monog. Soc. Res. Child Dev.*, Vol VII, Series #33, No. 3, pp. 11–85. 1942.

Hughes, B. O. "Variability Among and Within Individuals in Relation to Education," in *Merrill-Palmer Quarterly*, pp. 167–197. Spring 1957.

Johnston, F. E. "The Concept of Skeletal Age," in *Clinical Pediatrics* 1 (3): 133–144. 1962.

Johnston, F. E. and Malina, R. M. "Age Changes in the Composition of the Upper Arm in Philadelphia Children," in *Human Biol.* 38 (1): 1–21. 1966.

Kasius, R. V. *et. al.* "Maternal and Newborn Nutrition Studies at Philadelphia Lying-In Hospital. V Size and Growth of Babies During the First Year of Life," in *Milbank Memorial Fund Quarterly*, 35(4): 323–372. N.Y., 1957.

Krogman, W. M. "The Role of Genetic Factors in Human Face, Jaws and Teeth: A Review," in *Eugenics Review*, 57 (3): 165–192. Sept. 1967.

Lenz, W. "Chemicals and Malformation in Man," in *Congenital Malformations*, 2nd Internat. Cong. Publ. by the International Congress, Ltd. 1964.

Li, C. H. "The Pituitary," in *Sci. Amer.* Oct. 1950.

Malina, R. M. "Exercise as an Influence Upon Growth: Review and Critique of Current Concepts," in *Clinical Pediatrics* 8 (1): 16–26. 1969a.

Malina, R. M. "Growth and Physical Performance of American Negro and White Children," in *Clinical Pediatrics* 8 (8): 476–483. 1969b.

Malina, R. M. "Quantification of Fat, Muscle, and Bone in Man," in *Clinical Orthopaedics and Related Research* 65: 9–38. July-August, 1969.

Mann, H. C. Diets for Boys During the School Age. *Med. Res. Council*, London. Series #105. 1926.

Massler, M. and Suher, T. "Calculations of Normal Weight," in *Child Development* 16 (1–2): 111–116. 1945.

Meredith, H. V. "Length of Head and Neck, Trunk, and Lower Extremities of Iowa City Children, Aged 7–17 years," in *Child Development* 10 (2): 129–144. 1939.

Meredith, H. V. "Changes in the Stature and Body Weight of N. A. Boys During the Last 80 Years" (pp. 69–114, in Lipsitt, L. P. and C. C. Spiker, *Advances in Child Development and Behavior*, (I). New York, 1963.

Mills, C. A. "Climatic Effects on Growth and Development, With Particular Reference to the Effects of Tropical Residence," in *Am. Anth.* 41 (1): 1–13. 1942.

Morley, A. J. M. "Knock-Knees in Children," in *Brit. Med. J.*, pp. 976–979. Oct. 26, 1957.

Nicolson, A. B. and Hanley, C. "Indices of Physiological Maturity: Derivation and Inter-Relationships," in *Child Development* 24 (1): 3–38. 1953.

Olson, W. C. "Developmental Theory in Education" (pp. 259–274, in Harris, D. B., ed., *The Concept of Development*). Minneapolis, 1957.

Prader, A. and Tanner, J. M. "Catch-Up Growth Following Illness or Starvation," in *J. Pediatrics* 62 (5): 646–659. 1963.

Reynolds, E. "Differential Tissue Growth in the Leg During Childhood," in *Child Development* 15 (4): 181–205. 1946.

Robinow, M. *et. al.* "Feet in Normal Children," in *J. Pediat.* 23 (2): 141–149. 1943.

Scrimshaw, N. S. and Behar, M. "Protein Malnutrition in Young Children," in *Science* 133 (3470): 2039–2047. June 30, 1961.

Seltzer, C. C. and Mayer, J. "Body Build and Obesity: Who Are The Obese?" *J. Amer. Med. Assoc.* 189: 677–684. 1964.

Sevringhaus, E. (ed.). "Giantism and Dwarfism," in *Roche Review* 10 (8): 289–298. May 1946.

Shelton, E. K. and Skeels, R. F. "Endocrines and Growth," in *Ciba Clin. Symp.* 3 (6). Sept. 1951. Summit, N.J.

Simmons, K. and Greulich, W. W. "Menarcheal Age and the Height, Weight, and Skeletal Age of Girls Age 7–17 Years," in *J. Pediat.* 22: 518–548. 1943.

Simmons, K. and Todd, T. W. "Growth of Well Children: Analysis of Stature and Weight, Three Months to 13 Years," *Growth*, II (2): 93–134. 1938.

Sontag, L. W. and Lipford, J. "The Effects of Illness and Other Factors on the Appearance Pattern of Skeletal Epiphyses." *J. Pediat.* 23 (4): 391–409. 1943.

Statistical Bulletin, Metropolitan Life Insurance Co. Competitive Sports and their Hazards. 46: 1–3. Sept. 1965. New York.

Stoudt, H. W. A. Damon, and McFarland, R. A. "Heights and Weights of White Americans," in *Human Biol.* 32. (4): 331–341. 1960.

Stuart, H. C. "Findings on Examination of Newborn Infants and Infants During the Neonatal Period which Appear to have a Relationship to the Diet of their Mothers During Pregnancy." *Federation Proc.* 4(3): 271–281. 1941.

Tanner, J. M. "Human Growth and Constitution" (pp. 299–400 in *Human Biology*, ed. by Harrison, J. S., *et. al.*). New York, 1964.

Tanner, J. M. "Galtonian Eugenics and the Study of Growth." *Eugenics Review* 58 (3): 122–135. Sept. 1966.

Tanner, J. M. "Earlier Maturation in Man." in *Sci. Amer.* pp. 21–27. Jan. 1968.

Tanner, J. M. and Whitehouse, R. H. "Standards for Subcutaneous Fat in British Children," in *Brit. Med. J.*, Vol. i, pp. 446–456. Feb. 2, 1962.

Tanner, J. M., Whitehouse, R. H., and Takaishi, M. "Standards from Birth to Maturity for Height, Weight, Height Velocity, and Weight Velocity: British Children, 1965 (Part I)," in *Arch. Dis. Childh.*, 41: 454–471. 1966.

Todd, T. W. "Differential Skeletal Maturation in Relation to Sex, Race, Variability, and Disease," in *Child Development*, 2 (1): 49–65. 1931.

Vandenberg, S. G. "Human Behavior Genetics: Present Status and Suggestions for Future Research," in *Merrill-Palmer Quarterly* 15 (1): 123–154. Jan. 1969.

Yerushalmy, J. *et. al.* "Birth Weight and Gestation as Indices of Immaturity," in *Am. J. Dis. Child* 109: 43–59. 1965.

Zuckerman, Sir Solly. "Endocrines," in *Sci. Amer.*, pp. 76–87. March 1957.

ACKNOWLEDGMENTS

The illustrations listed are from the following works:

FIG. 1. H. A. Harris, et al., "The Measurement of Man," U. of Minnesota Press, 1930.
FIG. 2. Based on data in J. Yerushalmy, et al., Am. J. Dis. Child. 109: 43–59, 1965.
FIG. 3. Based on data in J. Yerushalmy, et al., op. cit., 1965.
FIG. 4. W. Lenz, p. 270, in "Congenital Malformations." N.Y., Internat. Med. Cong., 1964.
FIG. 5. Based on data from H. Stoudt, et al., Hum. Biol. 32 (4): 331–341, 1960.
FIG. 6. Stoudt, et al., op. cit., 1960.
FIG. 7. Stoudt, et al., op. cit., 1960.
FIG. 8. Stoudt, et al., op. cit., 1960.
FIG. 9. Meredith, Fig. 1, p. 90, in L. P. Lipsitt & C. C. Spiker, "Advances in Child Development and Behavior, I," 1963.
FIG. 10. Meredith, Fig. 2, p. 105, in Lipsitt & Spiker, op. cit., 1963.
FIG. 11. Fig. 38, p. 72, in N. Bayley & L. Bayer, "Growth Diagnosis," Chicago, 1959.
FIG. 12. W. W. Greulich & S. I. Pyle, Radiographic Atlas of the Skeletal Development of the Hand and Wrist, p. 187, Stanford, 1959.
FIG. 13. T. W. Todd, Child Developm. 2: 1931.
FIG. 14. N. Bayley & R. D. Tuddenham, Fig. 4, p. 41, in Adolescence, ed. N. B. Henry, Chicago, 1944.
FIG. 15. H. V. Meredith, Fig. 1, p. 132, in Child Developm. 10 (2): 129–144, 1939.
FIG. 16. N. Bayley & F. Davis, Biometrika 27 (Pts. I-II): 26–87, London, 1935.
FIG. 17. Based on data from W. M. Krogman, "Growth of Man," Tab. Biol. XX, The Hague, 1941.
FIG. 18. Krogman, op. cit., 1941.
FIG. 19. M. Anderson, et al., Chart I, p. 5, J. Bone Joint Surgery, 45A: 1–15, 1963.
FIG. 20. Krogman, op. cit., 1941.
FIG. 21. Krogman, op. cit., 1941.
FIG. 22. M. Robinow, et al., "Feet of Normal Children," J. Pediat. 23 (2): 141–149, Fig. 2, 1943.
FIG. 23. Robinow, et al., op. cit., Fig. 3.
FIG. 24. J. M. Tanner & R. H. Whitehouse, Fig. 3, Brit. Med. J. 1: 446–450, 1962.
FIG. 25. Tanner & Whitehouse, op. cit., Fig. 4.
FIG. 26. Tanner & Whitehouse, op. cit., Fig. 5.
FIG. 27. Tanner & Whitehouse, op. cit., Fig. 6.
FIG. 28. F. E. Johnston & R. M. Malina, Fig. 6, p. 15, Hum. Biol. 38 (1): 1–26, 1966 © Wayne State University Press.

FIG. 29. Johnston & Malina, *op. cit.,* Fig. 7.

FIG. 30. E. Reynolds, *Child Developm.,* Fig. 4, p. 200, 15 (4): 181–205, 1944.

FIG. 31. J. M. Tanner, Fig. 27, p. 385, in *Human Biology,* ed. J. S. Harrison, *et al.,* N.Y., 1964.

FIG. 32. "Hormones," by Sir Solly Zuckerman, in *Sci. Amer.,* March 1957, p. 76.

FIG. 33. "The Pituitary," by C. H. Li, in *Sci. Amer.,* October 1950.

FIG. 34. *Roche Review* 10 (8), May 1946, p. 290.

FIG. 35. Culver Pictures, by permission.

FIG. 36. E. K. Shelton & R. F. Skeels, *Ciba Clinical Symposia* 3 (6), p. 200, September 1951. Summit, N.J., Ciba Pharmaceutical Products, Inc.

FIG. 37. "Hormones," by Sir Solly Zuckerman, *Sci. Amer.,* March 1957, p. 81 © 1957 by Scientific American, Inc. All rights reserved.

FIG. 38. N. W. Shock, Fig. 13, p. 75, in *Adolescence,* ed. W. B. Henry, Chicago, 1944.

FIG. 39. Personal communication from J. M. Tanner.

FIG. 40. W. W. Greulich, *et al., Monog. Soc. Res. Child Dev.,* Vol. VII, Serial 33, No. 3, 1942, Fig. 1, p. 6.

FIG. 41. Personal communication from J. M. Tanner.

FIG. 42. K. Simmons & W. W. Greulich, "Menarcheal Age and the Height, Weight, and Skeletal Age of Girls Age 7 to 17 Years," in *J. Pediat.* 22: 518–548, 1943, Fig. 1.

FIG. 43. Simmons & Greulich, *op. cit.,* Fig. 3.

FIG. 44. Simmons & Greulich, *op. cit.,* Fig. 6.

FIG. 45. N. Scrimshaw & M. Behar, Fig. 1, p. 2040, in *Science* 133 (3470): 2039–2047, June 30, 1961.

FIG. 46. Scrimshaw & Behar, *op. cit.,* Fig. 4, p. 2041.

FIG. 47. R. M. Acheson, Fig. 3, p. 80, in J. M. Tanner, *Human Growth,* N.Y., 1960. Reproduced by permission of author and publisher.

FIG. 48. C. A. Mills, *Am. Anth.* 41 (1): 1–13, 1942, Fig. 1, p. 4.

FIG. 49. J. M. Tanner, *op. cit.,* Fig. 2, p. 50. Reproduced by permission of author and publisher.

FIG. 50. Tanner, *op. cit.,* Fig. 1, p. 48.

FIG. 51. S. Vandenberg, in *Merrill-Palmer Quart.* 15 (1): 121–154, 1969, Fig. 3, p. 125.

FIG. 52. G. Dahlberg, "An Explanation of Twins," in *Sci. Amer.,* January 1951, p. 49. All rights reserved.

FIG. 53. A. J. M. Morley, *Brit. Med. J.,* October 26, 1957, pp. 976–979.

FIG. 54. M. Robinow & M. Anderson, "A New Approach to the Quantitative Analysis of Children's Posture," in *J. Pediat.* 22 (6): 655–663, 1943, Fig. 1.

FIG. 55. Robinow & Anderson, *op. cit.,* Fig. 6.

INDEX